American Dietetic Association

GUIDE TO

PRIVATE PRACTICE

AN INTRODUCTION TO STARTING
YOUR OWN BUSINESS

Ann S. Litt, MS, RD
Faye Berger Mitchell, RD

D1406809

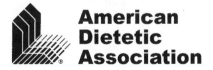

American Dietetic Association

Diana Faulhaber, Publisher
Jason M. Muzinic, Acquisitions Editor
Elizabeth Nishiura, Production Editor

10 9 8 7 6 5 4 3 2

Library of Congress Cataloging-in-Publication Data

Litt, Ann Selkowitz.
  American Dietetic Association guide to private practice: an introduction to starting your own business / Ann S. Litt and Faye Berger Mitchell.
       p. ; cm.
  Includes bibliographical references and index.
  ISBN 0-88091-347-9
  1. Dietetics—Practice.
  [DNLM: 1. Dietetics. 2. Private Practice. 3. Financial Management. 4. Practice Management. WB 400 L776a 2004] I. Title: Guide to private practice. II. Mitchell, Faye Berger. III. American Dietetic Association. IV. Title.

  RM218.5.L55 2004
  613.2'068—dc22

                        2004009032

Contents

Acknowledgments

This publication would not have been possible without the support of many individuals. We'd like to thank:

Amanda Archibald for thinking of us when the idea was developed.

Jason Muzinic, our editor, who calmly guided us through the process.

Pam Michael from ADA's Quality Outcomes Team, for her assistance in interpreting the technical MNT and HIPAA information.

The incredibly resourceful and generous colleagues on the Nutrition Entrepreneurs listserv, who were willing to assist other aspiring entrepreneurs by sharing brochures, business cards, and personal experiences to make this publication come to life.

Special thanks to Sandra Fishman, Cathy Leman, and Ann Silver for taking the time out of their busy practices to review our work and to Dina Aronson, Mary Ann Hodorowicz, Bruce Maliken, and Maye Musk for their willingness to answer questions and provide assistance as needed.

Our husbands, Dan and Andy, and our children, David, Jordan, Hannah, and Jessica, who saw less of us and more of "take out" than they care to share so that this project could be completed.

Reviewers

Sandra J. Fishman, MS, RD
Reading, Pennsylvania

Catherine E. Leman, RD
Glen Ellyn, Illinois

Ann M. Silver, MS, RD, CDE, CDN
East Hampton, New York

Foreword

Business owner, private practitioner, self-employed—titles that represent independence and responsibility. This publication, *American Dietetic Association Guide to Private Practice: An Introduction to Starting Your Own Business,* is a practical and honest guide for dietetics professionals considering individual ventures.

Starting a private practice requires more than clinical skills. Based on their individual experience, the authors provide a practical roadmap to evaluate the business and personal skills required before starting up a practice. This publication will assist practitioners in determining whether a private practice is right for them.

The authors also explore the multifaceted world of consulting for the practitioners, looking from traditional clinical settings to newer venues in the media and technology world. Information on marketing your practice, setting fees, networking—not only within your profession but in other businesses in your community—is invaluable to the neophyte private practitioner. Using case studies and practical experiences, the authors establish the fact for all practitioners that self-employment is a business, not a hobby.

My thanks to Ann Litt, MS, RD, and Faye Berger Mitchell, RD, for providing practitioners with sound information on the total concept of business ownership. Reading this book reinforces the fact that the field of dietetics is truly a "world without boundaries."

Marianne Smith Edge, MS, RD, FADA
President, American Dietetic Association, 2003/2004

Preface

When we were students in traditional undergraduate programs, private practice was just being mentioned as an option for dietitians. It was enough to pique our interest. When our careers started developing, we pursued the less navigated path. We each opened up a private practice in the 1980s and have stayed with it ever since.

We connected through networking and volunteering with our local dietetic association. We began meeting for lunch on a regular basis to brainstorm, to assist each other with case and practice management, and to help alleviate the isolation often associated with being a sole practitioner.

Two dietitians, practicing in the same community, working in similar specialties did not seem like the most predictable partnership. Yet we realized the power of working together rather than the fear of competition that often drives such partnerships apart. The need to network, the need to be connected to a professional organization, and the need to work together to promote our profession were some of the key factors that brought us together.

In 1992, we combined our experience and entrepreneurial spirit and created the Be Your Own Boss Workshops. Over a ten-year period, we conducted more than 50 one-day workshops around the country and delivered presentations on private practice to numerous state and local dietetic associations.

These practical workshops were designed in a "cookbook" approach to teach dietetics professionals how to start a private practice. This book is built around the same concept. It is intended to be user friendly. We do not want the reader to feel paralyzed by writing a business plan, overwhelmed by choosing a business structure, or inadequate at equipping the office. The book is designed not to intimidate but to encourage you to take the risk and enter the business world.

Use this book as your roadmap. It contains the tools you need to get started but is not intended to replace the advice of accountants, lawyers, graphic designers, or other professionals.

In private practice, you are entering the business world, with new barriers, goals, and issues. Your comfort zone as an employed health professional will be challenged. It will take time to get acclimated in this new world. To help you stay on course, familiarize yourself with the ADA Code of Ethics (reprinted in Appendix B), because one area that should never be compromised is your performance as a dietetics professional.

The primary focus of this book is starting a private practice. Initially, all your energies will be channeled into running the business and getting patients. When you become more established, you may see the need to diversify and include other work in addition to individual counseling. Occasionally, we take a detour and discuss various consulting opportunities for you to consider once you become your own boss. For some, private practice and consulting will be the perfect blend.

We have been fortunate to own our own businesses. We are glad you have decided to look at being your own boss, too. With this book, we hope to save you from making some of the mistakes we made. We also hope to provide you with the motivation and support you need to "just do it." The work is hard but the rewards are tremendous. We wish you good luck and a sense of humor as you set out to become your own boss.

Ann S. Litt, MS, RD
Faye Berger Mitchell, RD

Chapter 1

Private Practice . . .
Is It for You?

If you are reading this, you have given some thought to owning your own business. Many people dream about being their own boss. But it's not for everyone. Before you give up a monthly paycheck to follow your dream, read on. Carefully evaluate yourself as a business owner, your motivation for being on your own, and the pros and cons of private practice. Then, with paper and pencil in hand, complete the self-evaluation form in Box 1.1 (1), to help you determine whether this is an entertaining fantasy or a viable option.

BOX 1.1

THE SMALL BUSINESS OWNER'S APTITUDE TEST

After reading each question, simply circle your numerical response or write it down on a separate sheet of paper.

1. In the games that you play, do you play harder when you fall behind, or do you have a tendency to fold your cards and cut your losses?
   (5 if you play harder, 1 if you wilt under pressure)

2. When you go to a concert or sporting event, do you try to figure out the owner or promoter's revenues?
   (5 if you often do, 1 if you've never considered it)

3. When things take a turn for the worse, do you look for someone to blame or do you try and look for alternatives or solutions?
   (5 if you look for alternatives/solutions and 1 if you complain or blame)

4. Compared to friends and colleagues, how would you rate your energy level?
   (5 is high, 1 is low)

(continues)

BOX 1.1 (continued)

5. Do you daydream about being your own boss?
    (5 if you often do, 1 if you never do)

6. When you are faced with important life changes, do you worry and fret about them or do you look forward to them, do your research and consider changes exciting?
    (5 if you make changes after research and thought,
    1 if you are too worried to make a change)

7. Do you look at the upside of opportunities or consider the downside first?
    (5 if you always see the upside and recognize risks, 1 if you dwell on the downside)

8. Are you the happiest when you are busy or when you have nothing to do?
    (5 if you are happiest when busy, 1 if you are happiest when idle)

9. As an older child or young adult, were you scheming or have ideas about how to make money?
    (5 if always, 1 if never)

10. Did you work part-time or summers as a teenager, or did you head to the beach or pool over the summer?
    (5 if worked, 1 if beach)

11. Did your parents own a business?
    (5 if owned one for a long while, 1 if they never owned a business)

12. Have you worked for a small business for more than one year?
    (5 if you have, 1 if you haven't)

13. Do you like being in charge and the center of attention?
    (5 if you really crave those things, 1 if you detest those things)

14. Do you have a problem borrowing money?
    (5 if you don't have a problem, 1 if it's a huge problem)

15. How creative are you?
    (5 if extremely, 1 if not creative at all)

16. Do you have to balance your checkbook to the penny or is "close" good enough?
    (5 if "close" is good enough, 1 if to the penny)

17. When you fail at a project or task, does it scar you or does it inspire you to do better the next time?

    (5 if it inspires you, 1 if it scars you)

18. When you truly believe in something, are you able to sell it?

    (5 if almost always, 1 if never)

19. In your own circle, are you generally a leader or a follower?

    (5 if almost always a leader, 1 if almost always a follower)

20. How good are you at keeping New Year's resolutions?

    (5 if you almost always keep them, 1 if you never do)

Scoring the test:

80–100   Go for it . . . you should be a successful entrepreneur.

60–79   You probably have what it takes to be successful, but take some time to look over the questions where you scored low.

40–59   Too close to call.

0–39   Tests are sometimes wrong, but you are probably better off staying as an employee.

Source: Reprinted from *Small Business For Dummies, 2nd Edition* by Eric Tyson and Jim Schell. Copyright © 2003 by Eric Tyson and Jim Schell. All rights reserved. Reproduced here by permission of Wiley Publishing, Inc.

What It Takes to Be in Private Practice

What is your motivation for wanting to own your own business? Do you want to be able to spend more time with your patients? Do you want to have a work schedule more accommodating to your family? Do you want to make more money? These are all valid reasons for wanting to be your own boss, and they are all realities of private practice. However, not everyone is cut out to be an entrepreneur.

Before taking the giant leap out on your own, it is important to know what it takes to be a successful entrepreneur. There are personal and professional characteristics and traits typical of those who are successful (1–4). It is not necessary (or likely) that you naturally possess all these traits. What is important is being able to evaluate your strengths and weaknesses and to ask for help when you aren't capable of doing it all.

Personal Traits of Successful Entrepreneurs

In a 1994 article in the *Journal of the American Dietetic Association,* the seven personal habits of highly effective dietitians were identified (5). These habits are shown in Box 1.2. Understanding what makes a successful dietetics professional provides insight into the traits of a successful entrepreneur. Additionally, the following traits are recommended for those going into their own business.

BOX 1.2

THE SEVEN PERSONAL HABITS OF HIGHLY EFFECTIVE DIETITIANS

- *Be proactive.* Being proactive means taking responsibility for one's attitudes and actions. Being proactive means knowing when you have control over a situation and when you do not. Proactive people are not pushy. They are smart, value-driven, and know what is needed to get the job done.

- *Begin with the end in mind.* This is accomplished by starting each day with an understanding of one's desired direction and destination. Goals are selected by developing a personal mission statement that clarifies values and sets priorities.

- *Put first things first.* Know when to do the most important things first. Crises are prevented by keeping activities in balance and by focusing on important, not urgent things.

- *Think win-win.* The agreement or solution is mutually beneficial and satisfying to all persons involved.

- *Seek first to understand, then to be understood.* Listening is the key to building win-win relationships. Most people do not listen with the intent to understand. They listen with the intent to reply. Once people believe they are understood, they lower their defenses so real communication can begin.

- *Synergize.* Synergy results from appreciating differences, to allow creative cooperation or teamwork.

- *Sharpen the saw.* This involves creating a balance among the physical, mental, social/emotional, and spiritual aspects of one's life to have personal effectiveness.

Source: Adapted from Smith D, Rhoades P, Gines D, Tolman N. The seven personal habits of highly effective dietitians. *J Am Diet Assoc.* 1994;94:377-380, with permission from Elsevier. Copyright © 1994 American Dietetic Association.

Being a Risk Taker

It is risky to leave a reliable job where you are an employee with a regular paycheck, a benefits package, and a sense of the expectations for performance. Questions you never entertained as an employee will loom large when you are a business owner. How will you establish yourself in the community? How will you structure your day? How will you make money? These are questions you likely never had to consider as an employee, but they will weigh heavily on you as a business owner.

Many entrepreneurs are not natural risk takers. You can take actions to hedge your bets that you will succeed, but no matter how you package it, there is an inherent risk in moving from employee to business owner. To take that first step requires courage (6).

The Small Business Association estimates that 50% of small businesses fail in the first year (3). Minimize your risk and increase your chances for success by being prepared. Seek the advice of business advisors, dietitians who have gone into private practice, and friends who are business owners. Create a business plan and assess the environment to determine whether your business is feasible.

To lessen the risk, investigate the possibility of part-time employment while you grow your business. If part-time employment isn't an option, perhaps you will find it easier to "moonlight"—and build your practice by seeing patients in the evening or on weekends. Eventually, you will need to leave the world as an employee and enter the world as a business owner, and that will feel risky no matter how you structure it.

An entrepreneur will encounter many risks in the business world. That first step is just the beginning. Risk taking is a quality that eventually becomes part of your "job description." You will learn to tolerate risk and see it as energizing rather than scary.

Being Disciplined

To be on your own, you need to be disciplined. You will never again be asked to punch a clock, state where you are going in the middle of the day, or give an excuse for a day off. Without discipline, it may be tempting to not "go to work," since you aren't accountable to anyone but yourself and your patients.

By establishing workdays and hours when you will see patients, you will be imposing discipline and structure based on when you are most productive. Determine when you will do paperwork, whether you will go to your office on days when you don't have patients scheduled, when you will answer your phone, when you will read your e-mail, and when you will network. Potential patients will actually find this structure easier to work with, and it will force you to be more organized.

Disciplined practitioners will also need to plan events and schedule opportunities to stay current. As an employee, you had the luxury to educate yourself by attending grand rounds, to join journal clubs, or to benefit just from professional dialogue with colleagues. On your own, you will need to make the effort to keep your skills current. You may have to carve time out of your workweek to attend a meeting. You will need to set aside time to stay current by tracking issues online or by subscribing to and reading many different publications. You might also want to discipline yourself to regularly meet with colleagues just to "stay in the loop."

You need to be disciplined enough to take time off to attend a child's field trip, go on a family vacation, or just give yourself a mental health day. If you're not disciplined, you might find yourself doing paperwork in your office long after the "traditional" workday has ended. Plan a schedule to include free time, too. All work and no play will not make a productive entrepreneur.

Having Confidence

Some individuals are born confident and others need to find their confidence. If you are going to be successful, you will need to develop confidence and act like it was always there. The more successful experiences you have in practice, the easier this becomes.

Confidence is being able to promote yourself 24 hours a day, 7 days a week. If you aren't selling yourself, no one else will. Rehearse saying something positive about your practice, so when someone asks you what you do, your response can be a selling point (7). No one really feels comfortable relentlessly self-promoting. Be sure to assess the environment and determine when it is appropriate and when it just doesn't feel right to sell yourself. Refer to Box 1.3.

BOX 1.3
SELLING YOURSELF

- Tell people what you do in a way that they can fully understand.

- Exude confidence to persuade people to respect and trust you and the services you provide.

- Ask people for what you want—a raise, a promotion, or a contract.

- Be passionate about your business—passion sells.

Confidence means you are able to admit deficiencies and look for ways to correct them. A confident dietitian will readily refer a patient to someone more skilled in another area, send a reporter to a dietitian who might have more expertise in a particular subject, or call upon a Web designer to construct a Web site. Assessing your skills and determining what you are capable of handling and what should be delegated are also signs of confidence.

BEING ADAPTABLE

Being in business requires you to be a visionary. You must be able to spot nutrition trends in the marketplace. You don't need to be a trendsetter, and you don't need to compromise your beliefs. You do need to be open-minded enough to see the existing trends and recognize that your clients may want information on topics you don't agree with.

Being adaptable means knowing when to drop an idea that isn't going to fly, regardless of how much you like that idea. Moving on and getting over a failed project is part of being an adaptable entrepreneur.

You will meet many personality types in business. Although you are not required to become best friends with your business acquaintances, a flexible personality will enable you to keep many people on your side—an important asset in the business world.

BEING TENACIOUS

Entrepreneurs need to be driven self-starters who never give up. An entrepreneur will always see the glass as "half full." You will make many mistakes. Benefiting from those mistakes rather than feeling defeated and learning how to turn disappointments into learning experiences are important lessons for anyone in business.

Owning a business is demanding, exhausting, and of course exhilarating. To realize the exhilaration, you will need to be strong, to endure the emotional and physical demands placed on a business owner. It may be difficult at times to remember why you even wanted to be your own boss. Tenacity and drive are needed to energize and recharge—-even when you think you've made it.

Professional Skills of Successful Entrepreneurs

Unless you've entered the dietetics profession from a successful business career, there will be a new set of professional skills that you will need to develop. As a dietetics professional, you should be comfortable with your clinical expertise.

However, professional skills beyond your clinical training are needed to run a business. Gaining real world experience, whether or not it is clinical, will be helpful before you go out on your own. Most important will be your ability to assess what you can and can't manage on your own as a business owner.

BUSINESS SAVVY

Being a businessperson requires a transition in thinking. Dietitians are in a profession to help people. You will never leave that helping profession, but you will need to get used to thinking like a businessperson. What counts in business is the bottom line.

How you price your services is only one factor in determining your bottom line. Learning how to control costs, when to cut corners, and where to sink valuable dollars requires a business mind. If you are unsure, solicit input from colleagues established in the field already, other allied health professionals in practice in the community, and business organizations.

A unique aspect about providing nutrition services is that the public views nutrition and diet as familiar topics. Some may find it surprising that you charge for your services. Organizations, community groups, and even friends may assume this is a hobby, not a profession. It is easy to run into situations where you might be expected to give away your services.

Providing free lectures, volunteering at health fairs, or doing pro bono work at a local health clinic may be opportunities you view as important to promote your services. In business, however, you need to charge for your services to earn a living. You need to determine how much charity or "volunteer" work you want to provide and where you draw the line.

If you expect to be paid for your work, keep your rates and policies intact. Practice saying, "My fee for this will be," so that when opportunities present themselves, you will feel comfortable asking for a fee.

A savvy business owner learns to make decisions under pressure. In dietetics, you make decisions about patient care, so the foundation for decision making is in your training. Business situations may be unfamiliar, and you might have only your gut instincts to guide you at times. Thinking like a businessperson is a work in progress.

ORGANIZATIONAL SKILLS

Knowing how to delegate, organize, and multitask are tremendous business skills. A small business owner will be required to plan, organize, and implement everything related to the business. You will not have the luxury of a technology person to help you create a PowerPoint presentation, a secretary to schedule your appointments, or maybe even a janitor to clean your office. You will need to determine what you can do and delegate what you can't do.

You will need to multitask. Traditional multitasking or upskilling for dietitians has meant "the ability to perform more than one function, often in more than one discipline" (8). While this may come in handy, the definition of multitasking is quite different for an entrepreneur. You will now need to do things, such as send a fax, write a report, and schedule a patient, all at the same time.

As with traditional multitasking, the motivation will be for efficiency and to control costs. You must determine what you do best and delegate what you can't do on your own.

COMMUNICATION

Excellent communication skills are important in everything you do in life. In business, you must be able to communicate in a firm, positive way. You need to put a positive spin on your business as you communicate to the public. Being a good communicator means being a good listener, too. Whether you are communicating with a patient, a reporter, or an audience, you will need to become comfortable with the give and take of conversation.

The first introduction to your services may be the initial telephone call to schedule an appointment. Be sure your telephone skills are excellent. You need to be persuasive without making promises that can't be kept. Learn how to speak succinctly and effectively. If you have a receptionist answering your telephone, it is her skills that may be responsible for your patients making an appointment. Make sure she presents the style you want to convey to your clients.

There are many excellent resources available on how to communicate (9–11), which can be found in Chapter 9. If you are not a natural communicator, this is one business skill you will need to acquire to be successful.

CLINICAL EXPERTISE

Experience in clinical practice is a good foundation for any type of nutrition-related business. A clinical position in a hospital, clinic, or corporation can be a stepping-stone to opening up your own business. From each setting you will acquire skills and tools that will come in handy in private practice.

If you plan to have a medical nutrition practice, a strong clinical background and hospital-based work are essential. The experience you gain and the contacts you make while practicing in a traditional role cannot be replaced. If you plan to practice primarily in the areas not commonly classified as medical nutrition therapy, such as weight management, wellness, or general nutrition, you might find your clinical skills less important. Being attuned to the world around you, being well versed in consumer-oriented issues, and being a great promoter may be your most valuable assets.

Pros and Cons of Private Practice

When you are excited to leave employment and be your own boss, it is easy to see only the thrill and prestige of being on your own. Everything has positives and negatives. For most everyone in private practice, the pros outweigh the cons, but the cons still exist, and it is important to be aware of what they are.

Pros

ABILITY TO CONTROL YOUR SCHEDULE

One of the biggest draws to owning your own business is the ability to control your schedule. When you set your office hours, the days you work and when you take vacation are your choice. Take advantage of this flexibility by structuring your day around when you are most productive. If you are a morning person, set up early office hours. If you want to take vacation time during the busy holiday season, don't schedule patients during that time.

Private practice offers the luxury of flexibility. A private practice should allow you to practice when, where, and how much you want. You might be able to choose the hours you will see patients. You might be able to select an office location convenient for you. Be prepared to work more than you did as an employee. The difference is, you will decide when you will put in those long hours to have a profitable business.

BALANCED LIFE

Private practice appeals to many women looking to find the perfect balance of work with parenting. The image of a home-based office, close to the family, seems like an ideal solution. The reality is that starting a private practice and starting a family are both extremely demanding. They are not mutually exclusive, but both create stress and skills you might not be prepared to deal with. In an ideal world, you might want to have one or the other in place rather than embarking on both at the same time (12). The flexibility and ability to "call the shots" is an appealing advantage to anyone seeking more control over their personal life.

POTENTIAL EARNINGS

A dietitian in private practice stands to earn more than a dietitian working as an employee (13). Starting a practice, like starting any other business, is not a get-rich-quick scheme. Financial rewards take time. It is estimated that a new business takes three to five years to realize a profit (3). Starting your own business carries risks, but the benefits should include making more money than when you were an employee.

Once established, the dietetics professional may want to diversify her practice to include other types of consulting than just individual patient counseling. That way, the chances for financial and personal success are greater. You can diversify your practice and realize more profits by hiring other dietitians, writing articles, giving talks, or leading groups. Diversifying your practice will increase your profits and decrease the rate of burnout.

STYLE

Your practice will be a personal extension of you. What you say, how you say it, and whom you say it to should reflect your style. You are the boss. You only have to answer to your professional code of ethics, not the party line of the hospital where you are employed.

Regardless of where you work, you need to maintain a professional image. Think about your patients and your work setting. If you are renting space from a group of physicians, you may feel most comfortable wearing a lab coat. If you are working with a professional population, perhaps wearing a suit makes sense. In a health club, you may prefer to be more casual. Regardless of the setting, you will want to present a professional image.

PROFESSIONAL PRIDE

One of the most gratifying aspects of business ownership is the pride you have in knowing that you work hard for your personal and professional fulfillment. Success will be self-perpetuating. You need to be passionate about what you do . . . and sell that passion.

Cons

Anyone who is in business can speak to the pros and cons. Listen carefully. There are risks and struggles involved in being a private practitioner. For those of us who have been successful in practice, we can see the cons, but the pros far outweigh them.

DOING IT ALL

Nutrition counseling will be just one small part of your business. The challenges of learning many new things will seem overwhelming at times. You will be wearing all the hats to make a business work. When the fax machine breaks, when the scale needs calibration, or when the insurance company requests patient information, you will be the one responsible.

One of the downsides to having your own business is the push and pull to always be working. Work demands can place strains on personal relationships. Try to focus on the flexibility you have as a business owner. Remember your priorities when it comes to outside obligations, such as family versus work. You must prioritize the demands on your time. To accomplish this, you need to know that you will often feel that there is still work to be done.

You will carry all the responsibilities on your shoulders. You will take all the blame when things don't work out. This can be emotionally and physically draining. Recognizing that you can't make everyone happy is a reality of business ownership.

FINANCIAL CONCERNS

There will always be financial risk involved in owning a business. Cash flow may be a problem. To keep your business alive, you might need to invest your own savings, moonlight to have a steady income, or borrow money to stay solvent. In any situation, the financial arrangements may create stress in your life.

Financial issues ultimately affect those dependent on you as well. It is important to have the moral support of your family when you take on the risk of being in your own business. They may need to feel the sacrifice is worth it for you to succeed.

Financial concerns can become more intense should you become ill or need to take time off for other reasons. Whether you are ill, want to take a day off to attend a conference, or have to cancel patients due to inclement weather—these are all situations that will impact your bottom line.

Your income will be erratic. You eventually will come to know the normal fluctuations and patterns. In order to pace yourself, learn which months are busy and which are slow. Try to schedule vacations when your patient population seems more likely to be taking time off, too.

PROFESSIONAL ISOLATION

Going solo means just that. You are on your own. You must make an effort to network with others. There are ways to not feel isolated, but it is up to you to make that happen. Make a point to connect with other professionals regularly. Join relevant listservs, meet for lunch dates, or just go out for an afternoon with a friend. You will need to recharge to stay motivated.

Is Private Practice for You? A Summary

Here are the key points you should take away from this chapter.

- Personal traits of successful entrepreneurs include being a risk taker, being disciplined, having confidence, being adaptable, and being tenacious. You may not possess all these traits, but you need to be able to identify your weaknesses and supplement with professional help as needed.
- Professional skills for stepping out on your own include business savvy, good organizational skills, being an effective communicator, and possessing expertise in some area of nutrition.
- There are pros and cons to being your own boss. Be honest in looking at the whole picture before you jump into your own business.
- As dietitians consider private practice, they must carefully assess the environment and their own commitment. There is nothing more gratifying if it works. Being a successful entrepreneur should be financially rewarding and professionally and personally fulfilling.

References

1. Tyson E, Schell J. *Small Business for Dummies.* New York, NY: John Wiley and Sons Publishing; 2003.
2. Pinson L, Jinnett J. *Steps to Small Business Start-Up: Everything You Need to Know to Turn Your Idea into a Successful Business.* Chicago, Ill: Dearborn Publishing; 2000.
3. Small Business Association. Start up guide. Available at: http://www.sba.gov/starting_business/startup/guide.html. Accessed December 8, 2003.
4. Minter R. *The Everything Start Your Own Business Book.* Avon, Mass: Adams Media Corporation; 2002.
5. Smith D, Rhoades P, Gines D, Tolman N. The seven personal habits of highly effective dietitians. *J Am Diet Assoc.* 1994;94:377–380.
6. Dodd J. Look before you leap—but do leap! *J Am Diet Assoc.* 1999;99:422–428.
7. Lichten J. Selling yourself and your ideas. *Today's Dietitian.* 2003;5:18–20.
8. Visocan B. Upskilling and dietetics professionals. *J Am Diet Assoc.* 1998;98:1043–1044.
9. Boothman N. *How to Connect in Business in 90 Seconds or Less.* New York, NY: Workman Publishing; 2002.
10. Halli B, Calabrese R, O'Sullivan MJ, O'Sullivan MK. *Communication and Education Skills for Dietetics Professionals.* New York, NY: Lippincott Williams & Wilkins; 2003.
11. Carnegie D. *How to Win Friends and Influence People.* New York, NY: Pocket Books; 1998.

12. Stevenson L. A mother in private practice. *Today's Dietitian.* 2003;5:58.

13. Rogers D. Report on the ADA 2002 Dietetics Compensation and Benefits Survey. *J Am Diet Assoc.* 2003;103:243–255.

Chapter 2

Minding Your Business

As you move from being an employee to self-employment, you need to determine what you will call yourself. Are you a nutrition consultant, a dietitian in private practice, a writer, or an entrepreneur? Possibly you will be all of those titles and more . . . sometimes simultaneously.

The Internal Revenue Service (IRS) provides guidelines for determining whether you are an independent contractor or an employee (see Chapter 8). These distinctions are critical to determine your federal tax obligations, your Social Security and Medicare payments, and how and when to file your tax returns (1).

As you launch your business, you may decide to maintain your status as an employee but take on other projects as an independent contractor. Whether you are practicing entirely on your own or accepting one small independent project, the information provided in this chapter will help you understand the options for structuring your practice. It is important to be familiar with these terms before you sit down with a business adviser who can help you select the business structures most appropriate for you.

Advising Your Business

There are many types of business advisers available to help you do what you cannot do, do not want to do, or should not do. Since most of us have been trained as dietitians and not entrepreneurs, it is important to know when to ask for help. Spending money on an adviser who knows about small businesses will be a wise investment in your future. Following is a list of people and a brief explanation of how they might assist you in the business world.

Accountant

An accountant can advise you on your taxes, legitimate business deductions, suitable business structure, and overall record keeping. As your business grows, an accountant can also advise you on investments. It is best to work with an accountant who is familiar with small businesses. Be aware, however, that fees vary tremendously.

Attorney

It is advisable to consult an attorney before making any decision with legal implications, such as deciding your business structure, drawing up a partnership agreement, or signing a contract. You might also consult an attorney before signing a lease, negotiating a bank loan, or copyrighting written material. Be sure to hire an attorney who is familiar with small businesses and has fees in line with what you can afford.

Banker

Establish a relationship with a friendly banker. Even if you don't plan to take out a loan, a banker can often advise you on the best accounts for your business, lead you to credit cards with the most attractive interest rates, and even help guide you about accepting credit cards in your practice. A banker can also provide you with information on setting up individual retirement accounts (IRAs) and Keogh plans for small businesses. Best of all, the advice from bankers is free.

Business Consultant

A business consultant can serve as an overall adviser to your business. He/she may be able to guide you to an ideal office location, help you to project a professional image in the community, or offer ideas for establishing your business priorities. The best way to find an adviser is by speaking to others who have started a business. The Small Business Administration may also keep lists of people who are available in your community. Valuable business services are available through the Service Corps of Retired Executives (SCORE). SCORE services are free. You can find out more about SCORE at their Web site (http://www.score.org).

Marketing Consultant and Public Relations Adviser

♡ *Martin*

As your business grows, consulting with a marketing person or a public relations adviser might take you to the next level. These consultants can assist you with logo design, media contacts, or marketing campaigns. They are probably more helpful once you are off the ground and running. Fees vary tremendously. Shop around and be sure to get references from individuals with similar business goals.

Choosing an Appropriate Business Structure

Business structure is not a static concept. You might operate under more than one type of structure at the same time. What you may find to be an appropriate structure when you start your business may change as your business develops. How you structure your business will determine what you are entitled to deduct as business expenses, how and when to file your taxes, how to protect your assets, and which, if any, business licenses you are required to have.

There are essentially two business structures that you will choose from: those that fall under the category of "incorporated" and those that are "unincorporated." Sole proprietorships and partnerships are unincorporated businesses. Corporations, S corporations and limited liability corporations (LLCs) are examples of incorporated business options. The difference in the business structure determines how you will file and pay your taxes, the amount of legal paperwork you are required to complete to operate your business, how you will be able to raise money if needed for your business, and your personal liability (2–4).

Sole Proprietorships: Going It Alone

Sole proprietorship is the most common type of business structure in this country. Approximately 70% of all businesses operate as sole proprietorships (2). There is a good reason for this. It is the easiest and least costly way to operate a business. Should you decide to open your business tomorrow, you could essentially do that as a sole proprietor.

As a sole proprietor, you can operate under your own name or choose a fictitious name. (See *Naming Your Business* later in this chapter.) You can use your social security number, or you can apply for a federal identification number from the IRS by filing Form SS-4, Application for Employer Identification Number. Applications are available at the IRS Web site (http://www.irs.gov).

When you are a sole proprietor, you are the boss. You make all decisions about your business. You pay for all your expenses, you are responsible for all your debt, and you reap all the profits. Should you choose to stop practicing and close your doors, you can quite literally shut the door behind you and call yourself retired (or out of business).

As a sole proprietor, your business is not a taxable entity. You are responsible, however, for paying a self-employment tax. Your business expenses, profits, or losses are recorded on either Schedule C, Profit and Loss from a Business, or Schedule C-EZ, Net Profit from Business. They are then included with your annual individual tax return, Form 1040, and filed annually with your personal taxes. Depending on your profitability and your total household income, this structure could benefit you, because your business losses can offset the income you have from other sources, allowing your net taxes to be lessened. For further information on tax forms, see Box 2.1 (4).

BOX 2.1
SAMPLE FORMS FROM THE IRS

Federal Tax Forms for Sole Proprietorship

- Form 1040: Individual Income Tax Return

- Schedule C: Profit or Loss from Business (or Schedule C-EZ)

- Schedule SE: Self-Employment Tax

- Form 1040-ES: Estimated Tax for Individuals

- Form 8829: Expenses for Business Use of Your Home

Federal Tax Forms for Partnerships

- Form 1065: Partnership Return of Income

- Form 1065 K-1: Partner's Share of Income, Credit, Deductions

- Form 1040: Individual Income Tax Return

- Schedule E: Supplemental Income and Loss

- Schedule SE: Self-Employment Tax

- Form 1040-ES: Estimated Tax for Individuals

Federal Tax Forms for "C" Corporation

- Form 1120 or 1120-A: Corporation Income Tax Return

- Form 1120-W: Estimated Tax for Corporation

- Form 8109-B: Deposit Coupon

Federal Tax Forms for "S" Corporation

- Form 1120S: Income Tax Return for S Corporation

- Form 1040: Individual Income Tax Return

- Form 1040ES: Estimated Tax for Individuals

- Schedule E: Supplemental Income and Loss

- Schedule SE: Self-Employment Tax

Federal Tax Forms for LLC are generally similar to partnership forms.
Note: This is only a partial listing. Depending on your business, some forms may not apply.

Source: United States Small Business Administration. Forms of business ownership. Available at: http://www.sba.gov/starting_business/legal/forms.html.

Being a sole proprietor has some disadvantages. If you need to raise money to operate your business, banks may be reluctant to issue you a loan. You are responsible for debt incurred by your business. Should you be sued, it is possible that your personal assets will be at risk. Finally, unless you sell your business, in the event of illness, injury, or death, your business may come to an end. For a listing of advantages and disadvantages, see Box 2.2.

BOX 2.2
SOLE PROPRIETORSHIP

Advantages

- Easy to form and dissolve. Few if any legal documents required to set up shop. When you are ready to close the business, you simply cease to operate.

- Minimal paper work. Your state may or may not require you to register your business and obtain a business license.

- Taxed as an individual. Your business expenses and profit or losses from your business are recorded on a Form 1040 and filed with your personal tax form annually. Depending on your profitability and your total household income, this could be a benefit, because your business losses can offset the income you have from other sources, which decreases your net taxes.

- You must file a schedule SE, which is your self-employment tax. Not necessarily an advantage, but something you must do to be in compliance with the IRS.

- You are the boss. You make all the decisions related to your business. You don't answer to anyone else. You retain total control.

- The big bucks are yours. Once your business is profitable, you are entitled to all the profits!

Disadvantages

- Unlimited personal liability. You and your business are viewed as one by the legal system. If your business incurs debts or if you are sued, your personal assets, such as your car or your house, may be seized to satisfy a legal claim or business debt. You should have insurance to protect your assets, but it may not be enough to completely protect you.

- Funding your business. Banks may be less likely to lend to sole proprietorships than they are to lend to corporations. Funding may depend on your personal credit history.

- It gets lonely at the top. Being a sole proprietor can be isolating. You need to make an effort to interact with, and get input from others.

- Lack of continuity. When you stop practicing, your business ends unless it is sold.

Partnerships: A Match Made in Heaven?

A general partnership is when two or more people own and operate an unincorporated business. A partnership, like a sole proprietorship, is relatively easy to start. There are not any required legal documents, although your state may require a business license. Partnerships appear very attractive and can be beneficial to new dietetics professionals starting a private practice. Partnerships allow you to pool your resources, your talents, and your expenses. If you are just starting out, that means one scale, one set of food models, one rented office.

With a partnership, you can bring your talents together in a cooperative way. Perhaps one dietitian is a diabetes expert and the other has strong organizational skills as a result of her work as a chief clinical dietitian at a large teaching hospital. Combining these strengths can be very effective.

Reporting your income as a partnership is not as straightforward as reporting it as a sole proprietor. The partnership is not taxed, but each partner is required to report her share of the partnership income and deductions on Form 1065, Schedule K-1. (A sample of Form 1065, Schedule K can be found in Appendix A.) Many new entrepreneurs may require the assistance of an accountant to compile this information.

As with all business structures, there is a downside to partnerships. Partners expect much from each other. It is important to honestly assess and evaluate your partner as a business partner, not as a friend. You must understand each other's work ethic and share common goals and visions for the partnership. You must be explicit in determining what you expect from one another. If those expectations are not clearly stated, someone is going to be disappointed and the partnership will suffer.

Although you are not governed by legal documents, when forming a partnership (even with a close friend), it is highly recommended that you spell out all details in writing pertaining to the partnership (5). A partnership agreement should address the following:

- How you will make business decisions
- The purpose of the partnership
- Expectations of each partner
- How profits and losses will be distributed
- How you will terminate the business in the event of a partner's death, disability, illness, or desire to leave
- How money and time will be contributed
- How disputes will be resolved

Like a sole proprietor, a partnership faces unlimited legal and financial liability. That means each partner is responsible for 100% of the debts. If one partner incurs debt, the other partner's assets can be used to cover the joint debt. And regardless of your partnership agreement, a creditor may collect from the partner who is easiest to collect from. If one partner is sued, you are both vulnerable.

When a partnership is terminated, as when a marriage fails, you must clearly identify who is entitled to what. This can get very sticky if an agreement has not been developed and put in writing. For more information, see Box 2.3.

BOX 2.3
PARTNERSHIPS

Advantages

- Easy to form. Some states may require a business license to operate.

- Pooled resources and talent. Two heads are better than one.

- Little capital required to start and borrowing ability expanded.

- Taxed as an individual rather than as a business.

- Broader management base.

Disadvantages

- Think divorce. When you decide to split the partnership, it can be difficult to dissolve. Assets and debts must be divided.

- Like a sole proprietor, partners are personally responsible for all debts. If one partner is sued, both are responsible. The partner with more assets stands to lose more.

THE LIMITED PARTNERSHIP

Limited partnerships are formed when there are two or more general partners owning and operating a business and two or more "limited partners." A limited partner is an investor and is not involved in managing or operating the business. He/she is liable for their investment but not for the entire company. It is best to have a business adviser help you determine which type of partnership is most appropriate for you to form.

Corporations: Not Just for McDonald's

When small business owners think about corporations, visions of McDonald's, General Motors, or Kraft Foods may come to mind. However, even a single dietitian may become a corporation! In fact, many individual dietitians do incorporate, because of the distinct advantages.

A regular corporation is known as a "C" corporation. Corporations are legal business structures. Although they present more complex and potentially expensive documentation and rules for operating a business, many dietitians feel that the advantages far outweigh the complexities. Unlike the sole proprietorship and the partnership, a corporation is separate from the people who own it. That means that your personal assets may be protected from your business assets in the event that you are sued.

As a legal business entity, state laws govern a corporation. To be in accordance with such laws, paperwork must be filed and fees paid in order to conduct business. Generally, it is best to hire an attorney to assist you in complying with the paperwork generated from incorporating.

Once you incorporate, you will pay yourself a salary from the revenue you bring into the business. As with any business structure, this means that you will need to establish a business account so as to keep your personal and business funds separate. Corporations pay taxes separate from individuals. This may become time consuming and costly, especially if you pay an accountant to do this.

There are options available that make incorporating feasible for small businesses wanting to form a corporation. The S Corporation and LLC are two examples suitable for smaller businesses. An S corporation is created for the corporation owned by a single individual. It protects the individual's personal assets, but its taxing structure is similar to being a sole proprietor or partnership.

An LLC is a relatively new business structure and has only recently been available in all 50 states. It provides the business owner with similar protection from personal liability as a corporation, but it can offer a taxing structure similar to a partnership, rather than to that of a corporation.

Some states also allow professionals to form a professional corporation (PC) or a professional association (PA). PCs and PAs were created for lawyers, doctors, and other professionals and may be appropriate for dietitians in some states. The main advantage of PCs or PAs is that the professionals in the corporation are not liable for malpractice committed by others in the corporation.

There are no right answers about who should or should not incorporate or what type of corporation is appropriate. This is an important business issue that should be discussed with an accountant, an attorney, or a business adviser. For further information on incorporating, see Box 2.4.

BOX 2.4
INCORPORATION

Advantages

- The corporation is a separate legal entity, so shareholders are generally protected from corporate liability.

- Ownership can be transferable.

- May be considered more legitimate than a sole proprietorship and has greater ability to raise or borrow money.

Disadvantages

- Can be difficult and more complex to manage because highly regulated by government. There is more paperwork, creating additional workload.

- Formation of corporations can be expensive and time consuming.

- Incorporating may result in higher overall taxes.

The Business Plan: Planning for Success

Purpose

Whether you are driving from Miami to Dallas, cooking a Thanksgiving dinner, or planting your vegetable garden, you have a map, recipe, or plan to guide you to your goal. Without a plan, you don't know where you are going or how to get to the finish line. The same is true with your business.

Your business plan is your blueprint for success. Putting your vision down on paper doesn't make it a reality, but it does force you to focus on the essential information needed to run a business: who your target market is, what your philosophy is, how you will fund your business, what you will charge, and how you will market your business.

It is not only a good idea to write a business plan; it is essential if you plan to seek a loan from the bank. To get a loan from a bank, you must describe what your business is, your plans for managing the business, an plans for how the money will be used.

Don't be intimidated. Writing a business plan should not be an obstacle to starting a practice. It does not need to be a 40-page tome. It may be a simple document that helps you formulate your vision and pave the way to making this vision a reality. There are many models and guides available, so it is not necessary to start from scratch. (For listings of resources on this topic, see Chapter 9.)

What to Include

What you choose to include in your business plan is not mandated, but most business plans include the following information (2,6).

COVER SHEET

The cover sheet is a title page or cover sheet including the business name, address, telephone number(s), and contact information. A simple promotional description of your business should appear here, too.

EXECUTIVE SUMMARY

The executive summary appears at the beginning of the plan, but it is the last thing that you write. It should be no longer than a page and succinctly describes your business structure, the goals of your business, what makes your business special or unique, your expertise, and your financial needs. It should translate the excitement that you have for your business and encourage the reader to read on, especially if you are presenting your plan in an effort to borrow money.

TABLE OF CONTENTS

Like the table of contents in a book, this table of contents lists the information contained in your business plan and the corresponding page numbers. It is included to aid the reader.

ORGANIZATIONAL PLAN

This section outlines how your business is structured, where your business is located, and the equipment and resources needed to run the business. It also details what your services are, who will use your services, and why your services are important to the user. You might include an overview of your business, identifying your goals and objectives and why you are or want to be in business.

MARKETING PLAN AND ANALYSIS

The marketing plan and analysis is where you analyze and define your market. (Marketing plans are discussed in greater detail in Chapter 5.) You should include information about trends in the marketplace and how your services are impacted by those trends. Pricing of your services should be included in this section. You will assess the competition, detailing who they are, how you are different, and why consumers should choose you. You will also include your marketing strategy, which outlines the tools, resources, and techniques you plan to use for making the consumer aware of your services.

FINANCIAL PLAN

This section is critical to the business plan. It is here that you determine the cash requirements for your business, such as what equipment is essential for starting out. You will also project income and create a cash flow analysis. If you are just starting out, this section is based on projected costs and income. It will be important to speak to other dietetics professionals in practice to get facts and figures for compiling this information.

SUPPORTING DOCUMENTS

The final section of a business plan should include supporting documents. Documents such as your resume, contracts or leases, articles of incorporation, partnership agreements, and personal financial statements should be included in this section.

Conducting Business

The requirements necessary to run a business vary from state to state. Following is a summary of the general considerations and questions you will need answered before opening your practice. Your city hall, county court house, or state revenue department may have a comprehensive listing of requirements in your area. The local office of the Small Business Administration or the public library may have information and may offer classes specific to doing business in your area.

Naming Your Business

If you are operating as a sole proprietor or partnership, you can use your own name(s) or choose a fictitious business name. Fictitious business names are referred to as DBA or "doing business as." The process for naming your business varies from state to state. Naming your business protects your name locally, but it does not prevent someone in another locale from using the same name. It is necessary to file your business name both to protect that name from others using it and to use that name legally on your bank account.

Generally, if you are going to name your business, you must file that name with the county clerk or other local government official and be sure that no one else in your community is using that name. Publishing your fictitious name in a general circulation paper in the county where your business is located is one way to accomplish this.

If you are a corporation, naming your business is a formal process. When you begin the process of establishing your corporation and complete the required paperwork, the procedure for naming your business will be part of the documentation you will need to complete.

There are advantages and disadvantages to naming a business. Using your own name lends itself to better name recognition. If you are already established, this is a distinct advantage. Should you appear on television or get quoted in the newspaper, it is your name people will remember, not your business name. On the other hand, having a business name may give more credibility to your business in the public's eyes.

Licenses and Zoning

Licensing for dietitians varies from state to state. Consult the ADA Web site (http://www.eatright.org), to determine if the state you are conducting business in licenses dietitians. If you are operating a business in a state that requires dietitians to be licensed, it will be necessary for you to be licensed in that state even if that is not the state where you reside.

If you are selling a product, such as a book or pamphlet that you have written, it will be necessary to obtain a seller's permit or license. This is necessary for reporting sales tax information with your state. Seller's permits and the laws governing them vary by state. You need to contact your State Department of Revenue to obtain information.

Before you set up shop in your home, make sure you have checked out all the zoning ordinances for your neighborhood and acquire any permits or licenses needed to run a home-based business (see Chapter 4). It may be perfectly fine to operate a business out of your home, but you might be in for a surprise if you do not obtain that information first.

Insurance

As an employee, you might not have given much thought to the insurance your employer carried. As a business owner, you must consider several different types of insurance. There are many types of insurance policies. It may seem prudent to buy all, but the reality is you probably don't need all. Sit down with your business adviser and investigate what is essential for you to have as you start out. A brief overview of the common types of insurance policies used by most small businesses follows.

MALPRACTICE INSURANCE

As dietetics professionals become more integrated into the health care system and more widely recognized by society for their work, it will not be surprising to see more lawsuits filed. To protect yourself, you must obtain a malpractice insurance policy before you see any patients on your own. Read through (or have a lawyer read through) your policy. It may or may not cover all your new activities as an entrepreneur. Refer to the ADA Web site (http://www.eatright.org) for options available for obtaining malpractice insurance policies.

As an employee, generally you are covered by your employer's malpractice policy. As soon as you leave that place of employment, however, you are no longer covered by that policy. If you are sued for work you performed while employed and you leave that place of employment, you are no longer covered. It would be wise to keep a malpractice policy current.

GENERAL LIABILITY AND PROPERTY INSURANCE

You will want to obtain an insurance policy to cover the contents of your office in the event that they are damaged in a fire or flood or are stolen. In addition, general liability insurance should be purchased, to cover you in the event that someone is injured in your office. Be sure to ask your insurance agent about any other policies he/she may deem necessary.

HEALTH INSURANCE

If you've had the luxury of having someone else pay for your health insurance, you are in for a big surprise when you need to purchase it on your own. Health insurance is expensive! There are several options available for the self-employed. Professional organizations, including the ADA (http://www.eatright.org), offer their members group policies. Another excellent resource is the insurance available through the National Association of the Self Employed (http://www.NASE.org).

When you first leave an employment situation to start out on your own, you may be entitled to coverage through the Consolidated Omnibus Budget Reconciliation Act (COBRA). If you've been employed in an organization with 20 or more employees, your previous employer must extend your health insurance for 18 months. You are required to pay for this coverage. For eligibility requirements, consult the COBRA Web site (http://www.cobrainsurance.com).

LIFE INSURANCE AND DISABILITY INSURANCE

If you have dependents that rely on your income, it is a wise idea to investigate disability and life insurance policies. Disability insurance protects your earnings in the event that you cannot work, by providing a percentage of your earnings on a monthly basis for a specified amount of time. Life insurance policies provide your beneficiaries with a payment in the event of your death.

If you have had policies with a previous employer, it may be possible to take over the payments to continue coverage with those policies. Insurance policies are also available through many professional organizations, including the American Dietetic Association (http://www.eatright.org).

Contracts

A contract is commonly defined as "an agreement between two or more parties for doing or not doing something specified. Contracts define your rights and obligations" (7). As a dietitian in private practice, you may be presented with a written contract. An example of this is when you become a provider for a managed care organization, engage in spokesperson work for a public relations firm, or write a book. Other times you may choose to present a written contract to a prospective client. For example, if you are asked to provide weight management classes for a health club, analyze restaurant menus, or perform nutrient analysis for a small food company, you will want to have a clear understanding with the other party as to the work you are to perform and the compensation you will receive.

Dietetics professionals question whether they should hire an attorney to write or review their contracts (8). If you are presented with a written contract, it is likely that an attorney for the organization prepared it. If you don't understand the contract, you should seek advice from legal counsel familiar with service contracts. If you have decided to draw up your own contract, a good guideline is the following: the more specific you are about the material terms of the agreement, the more enforceable it will be.

Minding Your Business: A Summary

Here are the main points you should take away from this chapter.

- You can structure your business as a sole proprietorship, a partnership, or a corporation. Each business structure has advantages and disadvantages. It may be a wise investment to discuss your business with an attorney, an accountant, or a business adviser, to determine the most appropriate structure for your practice.
- You should write a business plan to determine your target market, to organize your business structure and funding, and to state the goals of your practice and how you hope to achieve those goals. A business plan is necessary to borrow money from a bank. There are many tools available to write a business plan.
- To conduct business, you need to explore the pros and cons of naming your business and the steps to obtain a business name, licenses and permits you need to obtain to be in business, and insurance policies needed and how to obtain them.
- Advisers to your business may include an attorney, an accountant, a banker, a general business consultant, a marketing consultant, or a public relations adviser. When inquiring about the services of these consultants, be sure that they are familiar with small business issues and that their fees are in accord with your budget. It is best to get referrals from colleagues in practice.
- You may be presented with a contract for certain consulting situations, or you may want to present a contract for your services. Depending on the specifics, hiring an attorney might be prudent.

References

1. Department of the Treasury, Internal Revenue Service. *Contractor or Employee . . .* Washington, DC: US Department of the Treasury, Internal Revenue Service; 1999. Publication 1779.
2. Pinson L, Jinnett J. *Steps to Small Business Start-Up. Everything You Need to Know to Turn Your Idea into a Successful Business.* Chicago, Ill: Dearborn Publishing; 2000.
3. Cross A. Practical and legal considerations of private nutrition practice. *J Am Diet Assoc.* 1995;95:21–29.
4. United States Small Business Administration. Forms of business ownership. Available at: http://www.sba.gov/starting_business/legal/forms.html. Accessed March 5, 2004.
5. Lesonsky R. *Start Your Own Business: The Only Start-up Book You'll Ever Need.* Newburgh, NY: Entrepreneur Media, Inc; 2001.

6. Eastwood A. Writing your million dollar business plan. *Ventures: Enterprising News and Ideas for Nutrition Entrepreneurs.* Fall 2001:17.

7. *Random House Unabridged Dictionary.* 2nd ed. New York, NY: Random House; 1993.

8. McCaffree J. Contract basics: what a dietitian should know. *J Am Diet Assoc.* 2003;103:428–429.

Chapter 3

Setting Up Shop: What Do You Really Need?

Before you see your first client, consider the impression you want to make on your clients or patients. You need to think through all of the furnishings, business machines, equipment, office forms, and supplies you will need to set up shop. Remember, first impressions are lasting impressions.

Finding Office Space

Before you determine *what* you need, it is essential to determine *where* you will do business. There are many options for securing space for your practice. Before you begin to look at office space, ask yourself the following questions (1):

- How much space do you need?
- Do you need a waiting area in addition to an office?
- Do you want to be accessible by public transportation?
- How much storage space do you need?
- Is it necessary for you to be in a traditional setting, such as an office building, or will you be comfortable in a fitness club, a storefront, or even your home?

It is prudent to keep business costs as low as possible when you are first starting out. Your market analysis will give you some sense of where you hope your clients or referrals will come from. For instance, if you are leaving a clinical position in a hospital and plan to receive referrals from the physicians you worked with in that hospital, your office should be in close proximity to that setting. (*Special Note:* If this is your plan, make sure you have not signed a noncompete agreement with your current employer before you select your location.)

Once you have determined the general location for your office, you then need to begin to explore your options.

Renting

Renting is the most traditional way to obtain office space. Check with commercial realtors, check newspaper advertisements, or ask around to learn of available space. Renting office space can be costly. You will be asked to sign a lease, usually for at least a year, and a security deposit is usually required. If you sign a lease for longer than one year, you could prevent rent increases for the duration of the lease. If changes to the space are needed, such as painting or reconfiguring your space, you can negotiate with the landlord. In some cases, it may be your responsibility. Remember, everything in the lease is negotiable, so if you want changes, it's worth asking for them (2).

Co-leasing

Still considered renting, co-leasing is basically sharing the office space. Two professionals join forces, allowing them to share rent and many other expenses. You can still expect to sign a lease, but you both have an equal voice in making decisions. It is important that you define all the parameters in writing before you enter into this type of agreement. The office must accommodate the needs of both professionals, and you must divide up the available time evenly. Your schedules must mesh. Should you need to switch days, you may not have that option. Even if you and your partner are extremely compatible, you still may want to invest in separate phone lines.

Subleasing

Subleasing is an option that works well for many private practitioners. Again, you are still renting space, but with a slightly different type of arrangement. It is often possible to find another professional with an office available certain days of the week or for specific times in a day. You may even find a vacant room within an office available to sublet by the month. Subleasing space in a physician's office can be an ideal situation. Most physicians do not use their offices one day per week and would welcome some extra revenue. There may even be extra space within the office that is not being used and is available, or the physician may offer you the use of his or her office. Although there may be no room for personalization, it is a great option when you are first starting out.

Another option is to sublet extra office space or a room available within a professional office suite or a health club. When subleasing, keep in mind that you may not be dealing directly with the owner of the space, so there are limitations.

The arrangement for determining rent for a sublease can vary widely. Some professionals have paid "rent" by giving the physician a percentage of total billings. The percentage the physician receives can range anywhere from 20 percent to 50 percent. This arrangement is not recommended, because it may be viewed as fee splitting. Fee splitting, otherwise known as kickbacks, is not advised. Recent regulations have tightened up on physicians benefiting financially from referrals to other health care providers. In certain situations, fee splitting has been deemed illegal.

Other "sublet" options include paying a set fee for the space by the hour, day, week, or month, depending on the negotiations. Another possibility is for the physician's practice to pay the dietetics professional a consulting fee for seeing patients. Physicians consider this a value-added service to their practice. In return, the physician's practice benefits from being able to offer patients more comprehensive medical care within the office; it also saves the physician valuable time by taking care of the patient's nutrition questions.

Whether you sublet or get paid a consulting fee, consider these variables when negotiating:

- Who will do the scheduling?
- Will the office receptionist greet the patients and provide them forms to complete?
- Who will do the billing?
- Can you use the fax, copy machine, and phone lines?
- Will business cards be provided?
- Who pays for educational materials?

All of these goods and services cost money, and therefore should be factored into the equation.

Other options to explore include the offices of psychotherapists, social workers, and other mental health professionals. Their offices are often available during their down times, and many of these professionals are used to subletting their space. Because you may be sharing space, this puts a natural limit on your available hours. It will require you to set regular office hours. Conversely, it limits your flexibility.

When subleasing, you still may be required to sign a lease, or at least have an agreement in writing. Some sublet situations will require a one-year lease. If at all possible, consider negotiating a month-to-month lease, with the stipulation of a two-month notice period. This will allow you to assess whether the arrangement is working for both parties.

In a sublet arrangement, make sure you are able to have all your supplies conveniently available for patient counseling. Having to wheel your scale and a cart containing all your papers in and out of the room each time you are in the office can quickly become tiresome. Consider installing your own telephone line if you have any concerns about sharing telephone lines.

Investigate whom you are subletting from. Be careful about associating with someone who may not have the best reputation. You do not want your practice to be impacted by another's poor reputation.

Other Possibilities

There are many places to find office space. Think of allied health professionals and the fitness industry, and don't forget to think outside the box for other possibilities. Box 3.1 provides some suggestions for your search.

BOX 3.1

POSSIBILITIES FOR OFFICE SPACE

- Physician's office

- Psychotherapist's office

- Dental office

- Occupational therapist's office

- Physical therapist's office

- Day spas

- Executive office suites

- Massage therapist's office

- Chiropractor's office

Whether you rent, sublease, or co-lease, there are many questions you should ask about the space before you sign on the dotted line. Refer to Box 3.2 for additional tips.

BOX 3.2
ISSUES TO INVESTIGATE BEFORE DECIDING ON OFFICE SPACE

- **Bathroom access:** Will there be a bathroom in your suite or in the hall? Do clients need a key to access the bathroom?

- **Signage:** Can you place your name in the directory, on a nameplate at the entrance to the office, and/or at the entrance to your individual office? Who pays for signage?

- **Security:** What type of security does the office provide? Is there a security person in the front of the building, a code for access, or must visitors be announced? This is particularly important if you will be seeing patients after regular business hours.

- **Snow removal and groundskeeping:** Who is responsible for the grounds around the office?

- **Cleaning:** Does the rent include a cleaning service?

- **Utilities:** Does the rent include utilities? Do they shut off after regular business hours? Is there a way you can pay to use them after business hours?

- **Kitchen area:** Do you want a small kitchen area in your office? If you will be there for long periods of time, you may want to have a place where you can make coffee or tea, refrigerate items, or store a microwave.

- **Parking:** Is parking available for you and your clients? Is there a parking fee? If so, will this deter patients?

- **Other fees:** Will the landlord make you responsible to pay a share of the building taxes and/or insurance?

- **Handicap accessibility:** Is the building in compliance with the Americans with Disabilities Act?

- **Furniture:** Is the furniture you see in the office now available for your use? (This is more applicable if you are subleasing.)

Home Office

The home office is clearly the most affordable option and the one that presents the least financial risk. However, some professionals find it difficult to stay on track when working at home.

If you choose to use a home office, make sure your office space is private. Ideally, you should have a separate office in your home where you see patients. Some professionals have been successful in creating home office space by partitioning off a section of a common room.

Consider how comfortable you feel having strangers come to your home. Do you have a separate entrance or will they enter through your front door? What about a waiting area—will it be your living room? Can you keep your house neat and quiet enough to receive clients in a professional manner? Some patients feel more comfortable coming to your home, whereas others feel the opposite. More advantages and disadvantages are listed in Box 3.3 (3).

BOX 3.3
THE PROS AND CONS OF SETTING UP A HOME OFFICE

Pros	Cons
No commute	Professional isolation or loneliness
Greater work flexibility	Hard to stay disciplined
Lower start-up costs	Difficult to have meetings
Patients relax more quickly	Patients are less comfortable in home setting
You can "squeeze in" home chores	Hard to set boundaries

Source: Adapted with permission from Nutrition Entrepreneurs, a Dietetic Practice Group of the American Dietetic Association. *Nutrition Entrepreneurs Tool Kit: Pros and Cons of a Home Office.* Chicago, Ill: ADA Nutrition Entrepreneurs; 2001. http://www.nedpg.org.

It is also important to set limits for yourself when working from home. You can do so in the following ways:

- Try to set a work schedule and stick with it. Make sure you leave time for your personal life.
- Arrange for childcare when necessary. It is very difficult to meet your clients' needs while working around kids' schedules.

- Take breaks throughout the day. Time away from your desk will ultimately increase your productivity. Get out of the office (house) at least once a day (2).

Having a home office may have some tax advantages. You are able to deduct your home office from your taxes if

- it is the *principal place* from which you conduct your business.
- it is used for meeting with patients, clients, or customers in the normal course of doing business.
- you have a separate building on your property, which you use as a home office.

Even if you do not meet the above criteria, you may be able to deduct your home office. Also, there may be limitations to the amount you can deduct if you do so. See your accountant or business adviser for further assistance with this matter.

Traveling Office

Some dietetics professionals can avoid the hassle of finding office space by making home visits. They simply gather their necessary supplies in a box and make house calls. This allows them to really see what their patients are eating, do pantry checks, and perform feeding evaluations. The downside is that they have to be extra vigilant in making sure that they have everything they need and that they are in a safe environment. It is also important to charge accordingly—travel time should be considered when establishing fees.

Outfitting Your Office: Assessing Your Needs

Take some time to imagine yourself going through a full day of work in your new office space. Visualize the entire process. What furniture will you need in your office? Where will you greet your patients? What will the patient do on entering your office? Will the patient need to sit in a waiting room to complete some paperwork? What paperwork will there be? How will you furnish the waiting room? Continue this exercise as you jot down all the essentials that pop into your mind.

Once you have done this, you will have a greater feel for all the essentials required to set up your office. Make a master list of what you need.

You can also ask yourself the following questions as a first step in preparing your list of essentials:

- Will you have employees working in the office? Some practitioners do have at least one employee, perhaps a part-time receptionist, so it is important to have adequate workspace. Sharing space with another health professional can raise another set of questions. For example, if sharing with an occupational therapist, will the office accommodate the other person's equipment and still leave enough space for you?

- Will clients be visiting often? Obviously, in private practice, the answer is Yes. Consider the image you want to project and furnish accordingly. Do you want to present a "medical" or a "counseling" image? When counseling, it is recommended that you not place a desk between yourself and the patient. The preferred counseling arrangement is to sit next to or across from the client, without a barrier. This fosters communication. If you are setting up another type of consulting business, the more often you plan to be seeing clients in your office, the greater the importance of projecting the right image with furnishings and decor.

- What can your budget accommodate? Clearly your available cash flow will determine your purchases. Set your priorities in advance, and stick with your decisions.

- What equipment must you have? You must decide what is essential to start with and what you can wait to purchase. For example, you must have chairs to sit on, but maybe you can wait to purchase a copy machine and make copies at the local copy shop.

Now that you have begun to assess your needs, the following sections will address further issues to investigate, before you decide exactly which forms, equipment, and supplies you will require.

Furnishings

It is important to purchase furnishings and equipment wisely. These items can be extremely costly, but think of them as investments in the success of your business. There are numerous sources for purchasing office equipment and furnishings, including your local office supply stores or national chains. (*Note:* If you are subleasing, you may need to work with the furniture provided.)

Search the Internet for additional sources. If your budget is really limited, you can check online auction sites or look for used furniture and equipment. Be sure to know your merchandise before you purchase anything secondhand. Evaluate the cost of the item new and the condition of the used product (2).

When furnishing your office, think of your clientele. Make sure your furnishings are comfortable to them. If you plan to counsel obese clients, it is important to select sturdy furniture to accommodate them, to make them feel at ease, and to avoid any embarrassing moments. If furniture is low, patients may have difficulty getting in and out. If you will be seeing families, you will need adequate seating.

If you will be dealing with corporate clients, consider an upscale look. Pattern your office after other corporate offices. If you consider yourself a nutrition therapist, look at the way psychotherapists furnish their offices. Many dietetics professionals who counsel patients prefer to have their desks tucked away in a corner as they sit with the patient in a set of chairs.

It is important to consider the type of lighting. Do you like overhead fluorescent lighting or would you rather use lamps?

Equipment

To determine which equipment to buy immediately, you may want to analyze how much the purchase of that particular product will increase your productivity and profitability (1).

THE BUSINESS TELEPHONE

Obtaining a telephone is not an option. Before you print your business cards, you need to obtain a separate telephone number. Having a designated telephone number for your business allows you to present yourself in a professional manner. Never use your home telephone line as your business line unless you are prepared to answer it with a professional greeting every time you pick up the telephone. Callers should always be greeted with your business name and/or the name of the person who is speaking (4).

Your business telephone should always be answered professionally. If you feel that it is important to have a real person answer the telephone and you cannot afford a receptionist or secretary, consider an answering service. Answering services, however, can mishandle calls, which results in client complaints. Carefully screen services and get recommendations from other business owners before selecting one.

Voice mail provided by your local telephone company is a good option. Most people are now accustomed to leaving messages on voice mail and will not be put off by having to do so. Voice mail allows you to set up multiple mailboxes. If you want to set up a separate mailbox for inquiries and one for scheduling appointments, you may be able to streamline your work. A standard answering machine is also a good solution. Many newer models also let you set up multiple mailboxes.

There are many options for obtaining a telephone system. Although it is tempting to go with the least expensive option, especially when first starting out, consider the potential for growth and look to the future.

One very simple solution is to purchase a cell phone that you carry with you. Most come complete with voice mail, call forwarding, and many other options you may need. Cell phones tend to have poor reception in certain areas, especially in office buildings. Make sure you have good reception if you are relying on a cell phone for your business. It is important to have clear communications at all times, and a cell phone may not be that reliable.

Instead of installing a telephone line in your office, you can have a second telephone line installed in your home and use either voice mail provided by your local telephone company or a standard answering machine. This allows you to be a bit more flexible with office space while you always maintain the same telephone number. For example, if you decide to sublet space on a part-time basis and eventually move into full-time space, you will not have to change telephone numbers as you move. Also, if you have more than one counseling location, installing and maintaining numerous telephone lines can become costly. The negative is that if you are counseling outside of the home, the telephone is in a different location. You will need to constantly check messages, and patients cannot reach you directly if they are lost or late. Some dietetics professionals remedy this by maintaining a home office line and carrying a business cell phone.

If you are renting office space in an office building and you want to install a telephone line, you will have to install a business line. Even if you are working from your home, consider using a business telephone line. Often, a business line comes with a free Yellow Pages listing. Consider also installing additional telephone lines for a fax and DSL Internet connection.

When setting up a home office, your choices for choosing a telephone may narrow slightly. You don't have the issues of multiple telephone lines for more than one location or moving your office. It is still important to have your telephone answered professionally, so consider an answering machine, voice mail, or an answering service. Decide on a residential or a business line, depending on your needs.

COMPUTER

A good computer is absolutely essential. You simply cannot run a business without one. If you do not already have a computer, assess your needs before you purchase. If your entire family shares one computer, purchase a separate computer for your business. This will allow you access to your information whenever you need it. It also lessens the risk of accidental mishaps and deleted documents or data. If you are not computer literate, consider using the services of a consultant to help you make this very important decision. (See Chapter 7 for more information on this subject.)

PERSONAL DIGITAL ASSISTANT (PDA)

A personal digital assistant (PDA) can help keep you organized. These items vary greatly in price, depending on their features. A PDA can substitute for a laptop on the road. It can keep your schedule and appointments, allow you online access to check e-mail, and maintain your contact list. You can even add software, such as nutrient-drug interactions and nutrition analysis, to a PDA, which can be helpful. Carefully analyze which features you need. You may find that you are paying for duplicate features, which is unnecessary. For example, if you are carrying a laptop to your office and have Internet access, you may not need that feature in your PDA.

FAX MACHINE

Medical practices are used to faxing lab reports and other medical information before patient visits. HIPAA regulations do affect your ability to fax information, and we will discuss this in greater detail later in this chapter. Still, a fax machine is an important piece of equipment in any office. As with the other equipment, fax machines vary in price. A basic machine may be all that you need.

COPY MACHINE

Copy machines can be quite costly. Weigh the benefits of having the machine available versus the time and expense of going to the copy shop. A copy machine might be a piece of equipment that can be purchased later, as your income increases. Another option is to purchase an "all in one" machine for your computer. These machines print documents from the computer, scan documents and books, and function as copy machines. This alternative can save you money, because you will be purchasing one machine rather than four machines.

POSTAGE MACHINE

Some entrepreneurs feel that it is essential to purchase a postage machine. Others do not mind the occasional run to the post office. If you will be mailing primarily letter-sized envelopes, you will need to purchase large quantities of stamps and have them available at all times. You will probably be mailing out reports to referral sources, thank you notes, bills, and occasional documents or handouts to patients. If you do not file insurance claims electronically, you will be sending insurance claims through the mail.

Additionally, if you are selling a product through the mail, a postage machine may make even more sense. In either case, you could start without one and analyze your turnaround time sending products out and how much time you are actually spending at the post office.

* * *

Technological gadgets designed to improve your efficiency continue to be invented. If you are the type of person that must be the first to have the latest technology, realize that you will pay a premium. That said, you should not ignore technology. In order to compete in today's market, you must figure out what technology is standard for running a business. Continue to evaluate new products, and make purchases as the market changes.

Business Forms and Supplies

You cannot run a business without certain forms and supplies. Some staples are necessary regardless of your setting.

BUSINESS CARDS

Creating business cards can be fun, frustrating, and exciting at the same time. Your business card is your first introduction to potential clients. A properly designed card becomes a powerful marketing tool and presents you in a professional manner (5).

It is possible to start simple with your cards. Initially, some dietetics professionals place their name, phone number, and e-mail address on their cards. There are many computer programs available that allow you to design and print your own business cards. This is an easy, inexpensive way to go when first starting your business. Many office supply stores print very basic, affordable business cards. Surf the Web for further resources. Many sites not only offer reasonable prices but also have helpful tips.

As your business grows and as your budget permits, consider designing a logo. A well-designed logo creates a lasting impression and definitely contributes to name recognition. The "Law of Seven" states that someone needs to see your name at least seven times before they will do business with you (6). Linking your name with a recognizable image from the day you start your business is great marketing.

You may want to hire a graphic artist to design your logo. What image do you want to portray? Are you more traditional or contemporary? Do certain colors appeal to you? Do you want two-color printing? If so, note that it will cost you more but may differentiate you from the crowd.

Once you design your logo, keep in mind that you will be using it on all your forms and marketing materials, including invoices, brochures, your letterhead, labels, and any other forms you develop (2).

Refer to Box 3.4 (5) for advice on designing business cards. Use the business card checklist in Box 3.5 (7,8) for tips on creating your cards. For examples of business card templates, see Figure 3.1. Although the cards are generic, they can give you ideas for layout and design. To give your card pizzazz, add your logo and/or some graphics.

When it comes to designing business cards, there are no rules. It comes down to personal choice and affordability. Determine which choices make sense for you in your situation, and have fun creating a unique card.

LETTERHEAD

Your letterhead should be designed as a package with your business card. Envelopes are also usually purchased at the same time. If you have not yet developed a logo, at least use the same font style and type size. You can create your letterhead on your computer with unique fonts. It need not be fancy, but it is important to convey a professional image.

BOX 3.4
DESIGNING YOUR BUSINESS CARD

- Keep it simple but classy. Use a legible font and nothing smaller than 10 points. Tailor the color scheme and graphics to your industry.

- Keep your card uncluttered. The most important information to include is your name, your company name, and your primary phone number. If you list multiple numbers (fax, cell phone, pager), put your primary number in bold.

- Put a photo of yourself on the card? Maybe. Business cards with photos may be less likely to be tossed or placed at the top of a pile of cards. If your first name is a unisex name, a picture can be beneficial. The downside of placing a photo is that the image, and thus the card, can become dated fairly quickly.

Source: Adapted with permission from Ratliff D. How to Use Business Cards to Land Your Dream Job. Available at: http://www.businesscarddesign.com. Accessed December 26, 2003.

BOX 3.5
BUSINESS CARD CHECKLIST

A good business card requires certain elements. Consider the following items:

- Name of individual

- Name of business

- Address

- Telephone number

- Fax number

- E-mail address

- Web page address

- Job title of individual

- Tagline or description of business

- Logo

- Graphic image(s)

- List of services

Some of these items are optional. Determine which ones are appropriate and most important for your business card.

Source: Data are from Bear J. Business Card Lesson Plans. Desktop Publishing. Available at: http://www.desktoppub. about.com/library/weekly/aa0828a3.htm and Ratliff D. Business Card Design, Marketing, and Printing Tips. Available at: http://www.businesscarddesign.com/critique.html.

FIGURE 3.1

Sample business cards. Cards designed using the business card template at DesignYourOwnCard.com.

Nutrition Services

Jane Doe, MS, RD
Registered Dietitian, Author, Speaker

555 Fictitious Street   (555) 555-5555
Suite 1200   Fax (555) 555-5556
Chicago, Illinois 55555   nutritionservices@fictitious.com

Jane Doe, MS, RD
Registered Dietitian, Author, Speaker

Nutrition Services

Your Sports Nutrition Specialist

555 Fictitious Street
Suite 1200
Chicago, IL 55555

(555) 555-5555
(555) 555-5556 Fax
nutritionservices@fictitious.com

Jane Doe, MS, RD
Registered Dietitian, Author, Speaker

Nutrition Services

555 Fictitious Street   (555) 555-5555
Suite 1200   Fax (555) 555-5556
Chicago, Illinois 55555   nutritionservices@fictitious.com

FORMS

Even if most of your paperwork is kept on your computer, forms are often necessary to gather the information needed to enter into the computer. It is recommended that you keep hard copies of most stored information on file. Forms you will need include the following:

- A *client or patient information sheet* or contact sheet. This allows you to collect necessary information, such as name, address, and phone number, on new clients or patients. Also consider having a space for the client's social security number on that form. Refer to Figure 3.2 for an example.
- A *fax cover sheet* is needed to send faxes. See Figure 3.3 for an example of a simple yet effective cover sheet that can be composed on your computer.
- *Invoices,* particularly if you are selling a product.
- *Checks* are also needed and sometimes overlooked. If you are writing your checks with an accounting software package, you will need compatible checks.

You can purchase standard business forms, such as checking and banking supplies, invoices, and statements, through your local print shop or office supply store, or from various Web retailers. As with all the business items mentioned, prices vary.

Remember to stock up on other miscellaneous supplies, such as pens, pencils, tape, paper clips, phone message pads, stapler and staples, etc. Make sure you have all the necessary computer and fax cartridges and paper you need. Always have extra on hand.

Patient Counseling Essentials

Patient counseling essentials can be placed in three categories: supplies, equipment, and forms.

Supplies

A well-stocked nutrition counseling office is different from that of any other health practitioner's. The tools required to effectively counsel patients and teach them about nutrition are quite unique.

FIGURE 3.2

Patient registration form.

Patient Registration Form

Name: _____

Home Address: _____

_____

Date of Birth: _____

Social Security No.: _____

Telephone No.:   Home (___) _____   Work (___) _____

Cell (___) _____   E-mail address _____

Occupation: _____

Employer: _____

Name of Person Responsible for Bill: _____

Address: _____

_____

Telephone No.:   Home (___) _____   Work (___) _____

Cell (___) _____   E-mail address _____

Referred by: _____

Reason for Referral: _____

_____

Current Doctor: _____ Phone (___) _____

Doctor's Address: _____

_____

FIGURE 3.3

Fax cover sheet.

RD's Name
and
RD's Logo

Digest This Information...

Date: _____

To: _____

Fax Number: _____

From: _____

Number of Pages (including this cover sheet): _____

Comments/Message: _____

_____

_____

Note: If you do not receive all pages indicated, or if there is an error in
transmission, please call: _____

Corporate Office • 128 Dietitian's Lane • New York, NY 55555 • (212) 555-5555

EDUCATIONAL MATERIALS

Patient education materials are crucial to imparting nutrition information to your patients. When patients walk out of the office with well-structured, clear, and pertinent educational material in hand, they feel as though they have gotten their money's worth! Many dietetics professionals create their own nutrition handouts and tailor them to their patient population.

When you are first starting your practice, however, time is an issue. You need to devote your time to marketing and developing your business. Why reinvent the wheel? There are many excellent materials available, so purchase what you need. ADA publishes numerous client educational items for purchase.

Many companies and enterprising dietetics professionals sell educational materials designed specifically for nutrition counseling. Food- and health-related companies, as well as other types of councils and agencies like The Dairy Council and the Food Marketing Institute, often provide free materials to dietetics professionals. For example, many of the large manufacturers of calcium supplements provide educational pamphlets about calcium. When deciding which materials you want to provide to your patients, it is best to review them and make sure the message agrees with your philosophy. The material might be free, but if it promotes an idea or a product that you do not fully endorse, then the cost is still too high. Chapter 9 provides a listing of resources for obtaining educational materials.

FOOD MODELS

Food models are a helpful visual aid for teaching patients about portion size. If you worked in a facility that provided food models, you may not realize how expensive they are. If your counseling style depends on them, your office will not be complete without them. Since they are expensive, research pricing carefully, and plan to work them into your budget.

Miscellaneous Supplies

Miscellaneous supplies for your client vary greatly. Some items that you may find useful in private practice include measuring cups and spoons (to demonstrate portion sizes), food labels or actual food packages, a flip chart for diagramming concepts to patients, and of course a well-stocked library with plenty of reference books. On the other end of the spectrum, you may also want to have coffee, tea, and water available for your clients. There are many variables to consider. Chapter 9 provides a more thorough listing of resources.

Medical Equipment

A medical scale is a wise investment. A balance beam scale is the most accurate. Patient population should certainly be factored in. For example, if you are dealing with obese patients, consider purchasing a scale that accommodates greater weights. A counter for the balance beam scale can increase the scale's weighing capacity to 450 pounds. There are also some accurate portable scales on the market, but they do not accommodate the morbidly obese. Practitioners who are sharing an office or who make home visits, however, find portable scales to be their only option.

Many practitioners find skinfold calipers to be a necessary tool, as well. If you counsel patients with diabetes, a blood glucose monitor will be useful. Contact the company who manufactures the various types of blood glucose monitors, and request a demonstration model to use in your office.

Client Forms

Nutrition assessment forms are essential. Some practitioners have more than one assessment form. They may use different forms for different types of patients. Some may shorten their assessment for managed care patients if their time with the patient is limited. Consider a 3-day diet intake form, a food frequency checklist, a food journal sheet (see Figure 3.4), a food history questionnaire and assessment form, a dietitian summary form (see Figure 3.5), a telephone intake sheet (see Figure 3.6), a progress note form (see Figure 3.7), and a release of information (see Figure 3.8).

A release of information form should be given to and signed by any patient who requires coordination of care with other health care providers. This form gives you permission to communicate with authorized health care providers regarding your patient's treatment.

SUPERBILL

A superbill is the foundation for insurance reimbursement. This form is a necessity. Dietetics professionals who do not file insurance claims for their patients present them with a completed superbill. The patient is encouraged to file the superbill with the insurance carrier for reimbursement. If you have the time, you can create a superbill on your computer. Collect samples from other health care providers as you visit them, and pattern yours after these samples. It is easier, however, to purchase superbills for a nominal fee (see Chapter 9). Chapter 5 details the issues concerning reimbursement and the private practitioner.

FIGURE 3.4
Food journal worksheet.

Date/Time/Where	Degree of Hunger	Before (Thoughts, Feelings, Activities)	Food Eaten	Degree of Hunger	After (Thoughts, Feelings, Activities)

FIGURE 3.5

Registered dietitian's summary sheet.

Registered Dietitian's Summary Sheet

Patient's Name: _____   Date: _____

Patient's Comments: _____

_____

Diagnosis: _____

Height: _____ Weight: _____

IBW: _____ Usual Wt: _____

Estimated calorie needs based on BEE:

_____

Pertinent medical history:

_____

_____

_____

Estimated daily caloric intake:

_____

% of daily calorie needs consumed:

_____

No. of excess/deficient calories per day:

_____

_____

Dietitian's signature

Manifestations

❑ Purging
❑ Laxative use
❑ Diuretic use
❑ Fasting
❑ Very low calorie intake
❑ Excessive exercise
❑ Bingeing
❑ Excessive calorie intake

Nutritional Status

Food Groups	Inadequate	Adequate
Milk	❑	❑
Meat	❑	❑
Fruit/Veg	❑	❑
Grain	❑	❑

Specific excess/deficiency:

_____

Plan

Education on: _____
Meal plan: _____
Refer to: _____
Follow up: _____
Letter sent to: _____ Date: _____
Patient's insurance: _____

Reimbursement: Yes ❑   No ❑

FIGURE 3.6

Telephone intake sheet.

Telephone Intake Sheet

Patient's name: _____

Parent's name: _____

Telephone Numbers

      Home: _____

      Work: _____

      Mobile: _____

Reason for referral: _____

Referred by: _____

Scheduled date: _____

Time allowed: _____

Requested

Lab work: _____

Growth chart: _____

Food diary: _____

Picture: _____

Policy reviewed: _____

Philosophy reviewed: _____

FIGURE 3.7

Sample of progress notes.

Page: _____

Patient Name: _____

PROGRESS NOTES

DATE	NOTES

FIGURE 3.8

Authorization for release of information.

Authorization for Release of Information

I authorize

_____

Name of sending person, agency, or institution

_____

Address

_____

City   State   Zip

_____

Telephone Number

to exchange
records with

_____

Name of receiving person, agency, or institution

_____

Address

_____

City   State   Zip

_____

Telephone Number

with regard to _____

Patient's Name

_____   _____

Signature of Responsible Person   Date

HIPAA Forms

Specific HIPAA forms are mandated by federal regulations. These forms, which inform patients of their rights to privacy with regard to their medical information, must be signed by each patient. There are two separate forms. The patient must be given a HIPAA Privacy Notice, which details privacy rights. You can download a sample of this form from the ADA (members-only) Web site (http://www.eatright.org/Member/Files/hipaa040203b.doc). This form can be found in the Appendix.

The second form, the Patient Written Acknowledgement Confirming Receipt of Privacy Notice, must be signed by the patient and placed in the patient's medical chart. A sample of this form can also be downloaded from the ADA (members-only) Web site (http://www.eatright.org/Member/Policy Initiatives/83_11022.cfm). The Patient Acknowledgment Confirming Receipt form can be found in Figure 3.9.

Patient Charts

Each practitioner has a preferred way of keeping pertinent information on their patients. Some use a manila folder with the patient's name on the front tab; others keep notes in their laptop. In your patient charts, you should keep copies of patient registration, insurance information, progress notes, payment information, and food journals.

FIGURE 3.9

Form for patient confirmation of receipt of privacy notice. Reprinted with permission from American Dietetic Association Web site. Available at: www.eatright.org/member/policyinitiatives/83_11022.cfm.

Patient Written Acknowledgment Confirming Receipt of Privacy Notice
[Print on clinic letterhead, if applicable]

I have received [insert clinic's name] HIPAA Privacy Notice.

_____(patient/client signature)

_____(date)

WAITING ROOM READING

Once you have all your patient counseling supplies, the last step is to stock your waiting room with reading material. Consider some health-related publications, but make sure the messages they give are consistent with your philosophy. For example, if a particular publication touts the latest low-carbohydrate diets and you do not believe in them, this may not be what you want your patients to read while they wait to see you. Having a daily newspaper delivered and subscribing to standard periodicals, such as *Time, Newsweek,* and women's and men's magazines, are always safe choices.

To assist you in setting up your office, use the checklist in Figure 3.10, to make sure you have covered every detail.

Setting up your office should be fun and exciting. This is the step that really seals the deal. You are in business for yourself!

HIPAA: The Bottom Line

HIPAA refers to the Health Insurance Portability and Accountability Act of 1996. The act establishes standards for electronic transactions and "Standards for Privacy of Individually Identifiable Health Information" (9). Trying to decipher

---

FIGURE 3.10

Checklist for setting up an office.

❑ Procure space

❑ Sign lease

❑ Arrange for painting, carpeting, construction work, or other changes to space

❑ Order nameplates for door and directory

❑ Purchase furniture; set delivery date

❑ Arrange for cleaning service (if necessary)

❑ Obtain parking space (if necessary)

❑ Obtain keys

❑ Notify security

❑ Order telephone line(s)

❑ Order fax line

(continues)

FIGURE 3.10 (continued)

- ❑ Order DSL line (or other Internet access)
- ❑ Decide on answering system
- ❑ Purchase cell phone
- ❑ Design logo
- ❑ Order stationery, business cards, announcements
- ❑ Purchase insurance
  - ❑ Malpractice
  - ❑ Liability
  - ❑ Theft and fire
  - ❑ Disability
- ❑ Purchase office equipment
  - ❑ Computer
  - ❑ Fax machine
  - ❑ Scale
  - ❑ Copy machine
  - ❑ Personal digital assistant (PDA)
  - ❑ Food models
- ❑ Set up billing/bookkeeping system
- ❑ Purchase or create educational materials
- ❑ Purchase or create office start-up forms
  - ❑ HIPAA Privacy Notice
  - ❑ Patient Written Acknowledgment Confirming Receipt of Privacy Notice
  - ❑ ADA MNT Evidenced-Based Guides For Practice (CD-ROMs)
- ❑ Purchase Office Supplies
  - ❑ Stapler
  - ❑ Pens and pencils
  - ❑ Paper
  - ❑ Cartridges
- ❑ Establish office policies—hours, fees, payments, schedule, etc.
- ❑ MARKET!!!
- ❑ NETWORK!!!

the regulations and figuring out how they apply to your practice can be quite confusing. In this section, we cover the most important facts, outline what you should do in your practice, and provide you with resources for more information.

HIPAA regulations specify that "Covered Entities" must comply with certain regulatory requirements. Covered entities are defined as health plans, health clearinghouses, and health care providers who transmit health information electronically (10). Exceptions exist for providers with fewer than ten full-time-equivalent (FTE) employees and those who do not transmit claims electronically (11). Solo practitioners not submitting electronic claims fall under that category and are therefore exempt from the regulations. Refer to Box 3.6 for more information (11).

If exempt, you must follow state confidentiality and privacy laws. To find out more about your state and local regulations, ADA has provided some information on the members-only Web site (http://www.eatright.org/Member/PolicyInitiatives/83_17935.cfm).

If you are still not sure whether you are a covered entity, or if you just want to cover all the bases, you can go to the Web site of the Centers for Medicare & Medicaid Services (CMS) (http://www.hhs.gov/ocr/hipaa). Click on "Am I a Covered Entity?" and complete the decision tools they provide. The CMS's covered entity flowchart is designed to help with this process.

BOX 3.6
HIPAA GUIDELINES FOR SMALL PROVIDERS

1. Does your office conduct *all* the following transactions on paper, by phone, or by FAX (from a dedicated fax machine, as opposed to faxing from a computer)?

   - Submitting claims or managed care encounter information

   - Checking claim status inquiry and response

   - Checking eligibility and receiving a response

   - Checking referral certifications and authorizations

   - Enrolling and disenrolling in a health plan

   - Receiving health care payments and remittance advice

   - Providing coordination of benefits

If your office does not conduct any of the above standard transactions electronically and if you do not have someone else conduct them electronically on your behalf—such as a clearinghouse or billing service—*you are not a covered entity and HIPAA does not apply to you.*

(continues)

BOX 3.6 (continued)

2. Do you bill Medicare and are you a small provider with fewer than 10 full-time-equivalent employees? Effective October 16, 2003, Medicare may not pay claims submitted on paper, with certain exceptions. One of the major exceptions is for claims submitted by "a small provider of services or supplier." The term "small provider of services or supplier" means:

   • A provider of services with fewer than 25 full-time-equivalent employees, and

   • A physician, practitioner, facility, or supplier (other than provider of services) with fewer than 10 full-time-equivalent employees.

If you do not meet the small provider exception, effective October 16, 2003, you will be required to submit your Medicare claims electronically. Once you begin submitting claims electronically to Medicare, your answer to question 1 above would be "no," and you would become a covered entity under HIPAA.

[*Note:* Small providers must comply with HIPAA regulations if they perform any of the following tasks electronically: submit claims, check claim status, check eligibility, check referral certifications and authorizations, enroll in a health care plan, receive health care payments and remittance advice, or provide coordination of benefits.]

Source: Department of Health and Human Services. Are small providers covered entities under HIPAA? Available at: http://www.medicarenhic.com/hipaa/downloads/smallhipaa_0703.htm.

HIPAA imposes certain obligations on covered entities with respect to their use, disclosure, and maintenance of Personal Health Information (PHI) (12). PHI is any information that connects medical information to a patient's name. Opinions may vary as to what constitutes PHI. When a patient signs his name on a sign-in sheet, is that PHI, or does it become PHI if the sheet lists "reason for visit"?

It is best to review HIPAA information on CMS's Web site (http://www.cms.gov/hipaa/default/asp), check ADA's resources, or consult with an attorney who specializes in HIPAA if you have specific questions. Answers can vary because you are dealing with interpretation of the law.

Depending on the size of your new practice (you may be flying solo at first), some recommendations, outlined in the article titled "Additional Covered Entity Obligations under HIPAA" (12), posted on ADA's Web site (http://www.eatright.org), may or may not be applicable (see Box 3.7). Research the material carefully.

These are the regulations, so how does this translate to what you need to do in your practice to comply with these laws? The following list presents some policies and procedures you should implement in your office setting (10,11,13).

- All patients must be notified in writing of your privacy practices at their first appointment. A sample notice of privacy practices for RDs in private practice can be downloaded from the ADA. Their backgrounder on HIPAA will link you to that form (http://www. eatright.org/member/83_12954.cfm).

BOX 3.7

HIPAA OBLIGATIONS FOR COVERED ENTITIES

Covered entities must

- Designate a privacy officer who is responsible for development and implementation of the covered entity's policies and procedures;

- Designate a contact person or office who is responsible for receiving complaints and providing further information about the covered entity's privacy practices;

- Train all the members of its workforce on the covered entity's privacy policies and procedures, as necessary and appropriate for the members of the workforce to carry out their job functions;

- Implement appropriate administrative, technical, and physical safeguards to protect the privacy of Personal Health Information (PHI);

- Enter into business associate contracts with persons that provide certain services to the covered entity, the provision of which involves the use or disclosure of PHI;

- Provide a process for individuals to make complaints concerning the covered entity's privacy policies and procedures;

- Develop and apply appropriate sanctions against members of its workforce who fail to comply with the covered entity's privacy policies and procedures;

- Implement policies and procedures that are designed to comply with the requirements of the Privacy Regulation (e.g., develop and implement processes for complying with a number of new patient rights);

- Develop a *Notice of Privacy Practices* that explains how the covered entity will use and disclose an individual's PHI, the individual's rights with respect to his or her PHI, and the covered entity's legal obligations with respect to PHI;

- Develop an authorization form for certain non-routine uses and disclosures of PHI; and

- Determine which members of the workforce need access to what types of PHI in order to perform their job functions.

Source: Reprinted with permission from American Dietetic Association. Additional covered entity obligations under HIPAA. [4/03 Prepared by Mintz, Levin, Cohn, Ferris, Glovsky, and Popeo, P.C.] Available at: http://www.eatright.org/member/policyinitiatives/83_11026.cfm. Accessed January 7, 2004.

- Each patient must sign a written acknowledgment stating that he/she received the privacy notice. You can also link to a sample of this form through the ADA Web site.
- The HIPAA privacy notice should be posted in your office (e.g., laminated or in a display rack) and on your Web site (if applicable).
- Business associates—computer consultants, attorneys, accountants, or anyone who has access to PHI—must sign a privacy contract.
- If your computer contains any patient information, you must have a password installed to access data.
- Fax and e-mail communications should have a confidentiality disclaimer on the bottom of them (see Box 3.8).
- Computer screens, if displaying patient information, cannot be visible to anyone other than yourself and your employees.
- Your file cabinets should be locked when not in use.
- You must request permission to leave messages on home or office answering machines regarding patient information.
- You should ask whether mailings should be sent to an address other than the home address.
- You must get authorization to submit PHI to insurance carriers. (This is often a state regulation and most health care professionals have been following this practice for years.)

Note that these are just some of the ramifications of HIPAA. The laws have been put into place to protect patient confidentiality. If you are a covered entity, make sure your office is HIPAA compliant before you open your doors.

Setting Up Shop: A Summary

Presenting a professional image is of the utmost importance. There are so many decisions you must make when setting up your office. Carefully assess

---

BOX 3.8

SAMPLE E-MAIL DISCLAIMER

This e-mail message and any attached files are confidential and are intended solely for the use of the addressee named above. This communication may contain material protected by any and all privileges associated with the provision of health services. If you are not the intended recipient or person responsible for delivering this confidential communication to the intended recipient, or if you have received this communication in error, then any review, use, dissemination, forwarding, printing, copying, or other distribution of this e-mail message and any attached files is strictly prohibited. If you have received this confidential communication in error, please notify the sender immediately by reply e-mail message and permanently delete the original message. If you have any questions concerning this message, please contact [insert dietetics professional's name]. Thank you.

the options, determine your requirements, and figure out which expenses can wait until you are a bit more solvent. Remember, though, you have to spend money to make money!

Some final notes:

- Before you see clients or patients, you must secure office space. Determine how much space you need, where you want to be located, and what type of space will work.
- Options for finding space include renting, subleasing, co-leasing, traveling office, or home office.
- Once space is secured, you must determine what furnishings, equipment, and supplies you need, and budget accordingly.
- A well-designed logo for your business card, stationery, and other printed materials creates a lasting impression and contributes to name recognition. Hiring a graphic designer is a wise investment.
- Why reinvent the wheel when you can purchase office start-up forms, patient counseling forms, and educational materials? This gives you more time for marketing, networking, and building your practice.

References

1. Mintzer R. *The Everything to Start Your Own Business Book.* Avon, Mass: Adams Media Corporation; 2002.
2. Friedman C, Yorio K. *The Girl's Guide to Starting Your Own Business.* New York, NY: HarperCollins Publishing; 2003.
3. *Nutrition Entrepreneurs Tool Kit: Pros and Cons of a Home Office.* Chicago, Ill: American Dietetic Association Nutrition Entrepreneurs; 2001.
4. Babener J, Stewart D. Setting up a home office. Available at: http://www.mlmlegal.com/homeoffice.html. Accessed December 23, 2003.
5. Ratliff D. How to use business cards to land your dream job. Available at: http://www.businesscarddesign.com/articles/jobhunting.html. Accessed December 26, 2003.
6. Bryan L. 10 steps to a stupendous business card. Available at: http://www.digital-woman.com/howto5a.htm. Accessed December 26, 2003.
7. Bear J. Business Card Lesson Plans. Desktop Publishing. Available at: http://www.desktoppub.about.com/library/weekly/aa0828a3.htm. Accessed March 3, 2004.
8. Ratliff D. Business Card Design, Marketing, and Printing Tips. Available at: http://www.businesscarddesign.com/critique.html. Accessed May 3, 2004.
9. Michael P, Pritchett E. The impact of HIPAA electronic transmissions and health information privacy standards. *J Am Diet Assoc.* 2001;101:524-528.
10. American Dietetic Association. HIPAA regulations for covered entities and backgrounder on privacy regulations and notice RDs. Available at: http://www.eatright.org/member/policyinitiatives/83-17993.cfm. Accessed January 8, 2004.
11. Department of Health and Human Services. Are small providers covered entities under HIPAA? Available at: http://www.medicarenhic.com/hipaa/downloads/smallhipaa_0703.htm. Accessed January 20, 2004.

12. American Dietetic Association. Additional covered entity obligations under HIPAA. Available at: http://www.eatright.org/member/policyinitiatives/83_11026.cfm. Accessed January 7, 2004.

13. Bodman S. Privacy, please: new rules may protect patients, alter hospital, office practices. *The Washington Post.* April 8, 2003:HE, 01.

Chapter 4

Money Management

The skills required to counsel patients in private practice or to work with clients in your consulting business are not necessarily the same set of skills needed to run a business. Traditionally, nutrition and dietetics programs do not require any business or management classes. To be successful in your own business, however, you must start thinking and acting like a businessperson. You need to constantly be aware of the bottom line. Often, dietetics professionals enter the profession because of a desire to help others. You can still help others while running your own business. You must, however, feel comfortable with charging people to help them.

You may have fantastic ideas and be an excellent counselor, but before you even hang your shingle you must have all your business systems in place. If you are not very good at money management, you may prefer to hire someone to do this for you. This will allow you to spend your time on other aspects of running your business. For example, if you can bill $120 per hour for your time and pay a bookkeeper $50 per hour, you come out ahead. From a cost-benefit standpoint, you may be better off spending your time on marketing, networking, and billing your patients while leaving the administrative tasks to someone else.

The downside of hiring someone to manage the business side of your practice, particularly when you are first starting out, is that it does cost money. Initially, most private practitioners prefer to keep costs as low as possible. Also, when you are first getting started, it may be beneficial to have a better understanding of the financial aspect of the business. When you do the billing and accounting and perform other financial administrative tasks, you get a clear picture of what it actually costs to run your business and to understand what is involved on the administrative end. As you grow, you can then hire someone as an office administrator or even a part-time bookkeeper, depending on your needs. Weigh the options, and decide which approach is best for you.

Office Payment Policies

Before you begin to see patients, you need to establish your payment policies (see Box 4.1). Will you accept reimbursement from private insurance carriers, or will you be entirely fee for service? Do you plan to become a Medicare provider? These options are discussed in greater detail later in this chapter.

BOX 4.1

OPTIONS FOR STRUCTURING YOUR PAYMENT POLICIES

You are at the point where you need to decide how to structure your payment policies. Here are your options:

- **Fee for service.** Some dietetics professionals have found it most beneficial to set their practices up as "fee for service" practices. The policy is simple. Payment is due at the time of the visit. You will provide the client/patient with a completed superbill. Explain to them that the completed superbill is the form that contains accurate diagnostic and service codes, so that they may file with their insurance carrier for reimbursement.

- **Accept reimbursement.** Many dietetics professionals accept insurance, which means they see the patient and then submit the claim to the patient's insurance carrier for reimbursement. Some carriers require that the registered dietitian become a provider in order to receive direct reimbursement.

- **Become a Medicare provider.** This is different from accepting reimbursement from private carriers. To become a Medicare provider, the registered dietitian must fill out an application to obtain a provider number.

- **Join Complementary and Alternative Medicine (CAM) networks.** Some dietetics professionals are finding it beneficial to join these networks. Referred to as "access programs," the patient—not the employer group or insurance company—pays the dietetics professional for the service. When the dietetics professional joins the network, he/she usually agrees to provide services at a discounted rate.

- **Become a Medicaid provider.** Medicaid is a program that pays for medical assistance for certain individuals and families with low incomes and resources. It is jointly funded by federal and state governments to assist states in providing long-term care and assistance to people who meet certain eligibility criteria. Since Medicaid is regulated and administered on a state-by-state basis, Medical Nutrition Therapy coverage varies by state. Further information on specific state regulations can be found at the Centers for Medicare & Medicaid Services Web site (http://www.cms.hhs.gov/medicaid/stateplans).

Once you set your office payment policies, you must clearly tell your patients what they are before their first visit. You should present your policies in writing at the time of their first appointment. Each new patient should sign a form stating that they have read and understand the policies and that they are responsible for payment. Inform the patient that payment is collected at the time of the visit. Then, patients know what to expect.

There may be situations, even when your policy is fee for service, where you have to send bills. Be sure to send out your bills in a timely manner at the end of each month. Usually you can minimize the quantities of the bills you send out by collecting payment after each visit, but there will always be exceptions. It is often difficult to get payment at the visit from teenagers and young adults whose parents are paying the bills.

Collection of Overdue Payments

You must have a policy for collections for those times when payment is not made in response to the initial invoice. How will you collect money from past due accounts? Begin with a friendly phone call or face-to-face reminder to people who owe you money. Most computer-generated invoices can be set up to automatically print a "past due" statement on the bottom of bills sent. When these approaches do not prompt action, consider sending a letter on your letterhead requesting payment within ten business days. You can state "if payment is not received within 10 business days of receipt of this letter, you will be contacted by our collection agency." In most cases, the letter will prompt payment. If not, depending on the size of the debt, it may be worthwhile to enlist the services of a collection agency. Some agencies retain a percentage of the total sum recovered; others charge a flat fee for each recovered account. To locate a collection agency, ask colleagues for recommendations or search the Internet.

Consider having a policy in place for handling returned checks. Determine what your bank charges you for returned checks, then work that charge into your fee structure. It is important to place this information on your new patient information sheet and/or post a sign in the waiting room. One great way to avoid returned checks and overdue accounts is to accept credit cards. This can also greatly reduce your accounts receivable (1).

Accepting Credit Cards

Before determining whether accepting credit cards is a viable option for you, it is necessary to do some research. The costs to the business owner are highly variable, so it is best to shop around. Often the credit card company will ask you to give an estimate of your expected monthly charges before quoting rates. A higher sales volume will generally provide you with lower monthly fees. Box 4.2 lists the options to evaluate before deciding which credit card processing company to go with.

BOX 4.2

CRITERIA TO INVESTIGATE WHEN CHOOSING A CREDIT CARD PROCESSING COMPANY

- Purchasing vs. leasing equipment

- Processing via the Web

- Is there a monthly minimum?

- Is there a monthly statement fee?

- Is there an enrollment fee?

- Is there a setup fee?

- What is the transaction fee?

  ▪ 5 to 30 cents per transaction or

  ▪ % of the transaction fee

- How long do you contract for?

Missed Appointments

Many practitioners have a 24- or 48-hour cancellation policy. They inform patients that they will be charged for missed appointments. Generally, you cannot enforce this policy for first-time appointments. If you inform each patient at the time they make their follow-up appointment of this policy, you can collect for missed appointments. **Important Note:** An exception exists for Medicare Part B covered medical nutrition therapy services. Providers cannot bill Medicare for covered services (such as diabetes and nondialysis kidney disease) that were not provided. There may be similar exceptions for other insurance carriers. Consult the guidelines of each particular carrier.

If you accept credit cards, you can have each patient's credit card number on file and bill for missed appointments. This policy should be printed on your patient information sheet and presented in writing along with your other payment policies at the first visit. Some practitioners find it helpful to have their policy printed on the bottom of an appointment card.

Setting Fees

One of the most burning questions from aspiring entrepreneurs is "How much should I charge?" Many factors must be considered when setting fees. There are a few formulas that will be addressed later in this chapter, but there is not a hard and fast rule regarding the setting of fees. Often it may seem a bit arbitrary.

Costs can be broken down into fixed costs and variable costs. Fixed costs are expenses you incur regardless of how many clients or patients you see. Examples of fixed costs include your rent, phone bill, insurances, and Internet service charges.

Variable costs, on the other hand, are costs directly associated with each patient or client. For example, each patient requires a file for his chart, certain copies of registration papers, and patient education materials. The more patients you see, the more of these items you must purchase, and the greater the costs.

Before setting your fees, make a list of all the fixed costs you think you will incur. Then, figure what the variable costs will be, to come up with a *per patient* cost.

Key Factors to Consider

When setting fees, consider the following factors.

SALARY

Determine your desired annual income (it is important to be realistic) as a starting point. Do you want to earn about the same amount of money that you earned in your previous job and reap the benefits of being self-employed? Or, is your goal to earn more than you previously earned? Either way, there must be some tangible benefit to having your own business.

BENEFITS

It is very important to factor in the cost of replacing lost benefits when setting your fees. Benefits usually provided by employers include health, life, disability, and other forms of insurance, as well as 401-K, profit-sharing, or pension plans. You will now have to pay for these benefits.

SELF-EMPLOYMENT TAXES

Another cost that is very significant and should not be overlooked is your half of the Federal Insurance Contributions Act (FICA) tax. Each of the FICA taxes is imposed at a single flat rate. Currently, the Social Security tax rate for employees is 6.2% and the Medicare tax rate is 1.45%, which accounts for 7.65% of your gross income. Because the employer is required to match this tax, a self-employed person is considered both employer and employee. The 6.2% becomes 12.4%, and the 1.45% becomes 2.9%. As a business owner, you now pay a whopping total of 15.3% of your income in FICA to the federal government.

BUSINESS AND OFFICE EXPENSES

Business and office expenses are often referred to as overhead costs. When first starting out, you should be somewhat frugal, as long as you are not so restrictive that you neglect to have necessary supplies and equipment to do the job properly. For a complete listing of the necessary office supplies and equipment you will need, turn to Chapter 3.

TIME

You also need to consider your time when setting your fees. In a service industry you are billing for your time. There are many things to consider. Determine your salable time—how much time can you really work, or, more specifically, how many hours can you actually bill? Again, it is important to be realistic in your estimates.

You may like to work a lot of hours. Certainly, this is great if that's your style. Elaine Biech, author of *The Business of Consulting: The Basics and Beyond,* estimates that two to three billable days is a realistic estimate (2). Psychotherapists, on the other hand, consider 25 to 30 patient-hours a full-time load.

Vacation time, sick days, holiday, and personal time should be built into your formula. Include at least 2 weeks of holiday time, 2 weeks sick or personal time, and 3 weeks vacation (3). Consider your nonbillable time, which always seems to amount to more than you may think. This is the time spent on administrative work, such as returning and making phone calls, writing letters, checking e-mails, writing and placing advertisements, paying bills, sending bills, and other accounting.

MISCELLANEOUS CONSIDERATIONS

Think about how much time you will be spending on marketing, networking, and continuing education, whether it is attending seminars, doing research in your office, or catching up by reading journal articles. A very simple formula for setting fees appears in Box 4.3 (4).

BOX 4.3

AXELROD'S FORMULA FOR SETTING CONSULTING FEES

How to charge to earn $100,000:

$100,000 income divided by 200 days	= $500 per day base rate
$500 per day base rate + $500 per day for overhead	= $1,000 per day
$1,000 per day + 25% add-on for profit	= $1,250 per day
Daily Consulting Rate	**= $1,250 per day**

Source: Reprinted with permission from Axelrod M. The Consulting Process: Setting Fees. Available at: http://www.thenewgame.com/axelrodlearning/consultingprocess.html. Accessed November 6, 2003.

Another simple rule from Elaine Biech is to apply the "three times" rule to calculate the ballpark amount you will need to bill to meet operating expenses. Triple your desired income to determine how much you need to bill annually (2). For example, to earn $50,000 a year, she estimates you will need to bill $150,000.

Setting Fees for Private Patient Counseling

If you are setting fees for private patient counseling, there are even more elements that can affect your pricing.

REIMBURSEMENT POLICIES

Reimbursement policies may have an impact on how you structure your fees. Handling insurance claims does increase the overhead for a practice. It takes more administrative time to check on eligibility and referral numbers, to file the claims, and to resubmit the claims if they have been rejected. Often there is a lag time between the time of filing and the time of getting paid. Because of the increased administrative time required, estimates for physician's practices for the overhead for handling insurance claims range from an extra $5 *per claim* to $30 *per 10 minutes*. It is probably comparable for dietitian's practices (5).

WHAT THE MARKET WILL BEAR

Although it is not recommended that you call other dietetics professionals to ascertain what they are charging for the same services, it is acceptable to ask consumers who have used similar services what they have paid and what they would be willing to pay. It is a *potential* violation of the federal antitrust laws to discuss fees for professional services. If dietitians were to *make an agreement* on price and determine what to charge, that would be a violation of the law. Antitrust attorneys advise health care professionals to avoid discussing fees with each other, to avoid any hint of impropriety (5).

A simple way to judge whether the market will bear your price is to try to gauge the reaction people have when you state your price. If most prospective patients do not balk and schedule an appointment, you know you are on target. If you get a large number of excuses or people saying they will call back, you may be too high.

Consider your *perceived* value. If your rates are consistently lower than others providing the same service, you may lose clients, because they feel you are not the best. On the other hand, professionals demanding the highest rates tend to have the reputation, experience, and higher levels of specialty that enable them to do so.

MISCELLANEOUS CONSIDERATIONS

Although it is a questionable practice to routinely charge service patients less than insurance patients (i.e., a cash discount), it is acceptable to occasionally discount your fees to a needy or indigent patient (5). You must determine how often you can afford to do this. You may also consider bartering for services, charging differently for home visits, or offering a discount for couples. If not dealing with reimbursement at all, you may want to offer different fee schedules for day versus night visits. Weekend hours could bring premium rates. You may also want to offer a family rate.

In general, you will have at least two levels of service—an initial assessment and a follow-up. According to ADA's MNT Evidence-Based Guides for Practice, the initial visit is 60 to 90 minutes long and follow up visits are 30 to 45 minutes. Some dietetics professionals take an hour and a half for an initial assessment. Set your fees accordingly, but you should consider whether seeing two patients in one hour requires more administrative time than seeing one. If so, it may be appropriate to set your half-hour fees to account for these increased costs.

When setting fees, be careful that you do not start too low. It becomes difficult to catch up. You can only raise your rates incrementally at any given time. For example, raising your follow-up rate from $30 to $60 represents a 100% increase. That increase would not be palatable to your existing patients. Take your time and carefully consider all the above-mentioned variables when setting fees.

Setting Fees for Contract Work

Setting fees for contract work or classes requires considering other variables that may be specific to the type of job. With this in mind, do not forget to factor in the following.

TRAVEL TIME

There may be time when you need to travel farther than the normal commuting distance. If you must travel to another city, take time off from another job, and/or spend the night, this should impact your rates significantly. Figure 4.1 (see page 76) provides an example of how to charge for travel time and other expenses incurred.

PREPARATION TIME

Preparation time is a significant factor in the equation. If you need to analyze recipes, go shopping, prepare food or handouts, or do any research, your fees should reflect this.

DUPLICATING COSTS

If you provide handouts or if you need to make copies for your own use in a project, don't forget to factor in duplicating costs. If you do not have your own copy machine, the cost of copies can quickly add up. When you do provide

---

FIGURE 4.1

Sample invoice.

[Letterhead/logo]

INVOICE

Client name

Client address

Date

Supplies for interview: receipts attached $_____

Radio interview (includes travel to/from radio station)
    2 hours @ $_____/hour $_____

Television interview—Boston, [date]
    1 day @ $_____/day $_____

Hotel expenses: receipts attached
    Boston, [date] $_____

Travel expenses: receipts attached
    Airfare $_____
    Taxi to and from airport $_____

Total $_____

---

handouts, consider negotiating to have the client make the copies. To do this, you must be prepared in advance, so you can get your handouts to the client. If you are the type who likes to make last-minute changes before you give a presentation, this may not work for you.

LENGTH OF THE JOB

The duration of the job is another important consideration when setting fees. How many hours is the client committing to? If you are signing a contract to provide services for a few months' time or more, you can probably afford to offer a slightly lower rate. A stable source of income, paired with a steady job reducing your marketing efforts, will allow for this.

PROJECT FEE VS HOURLY FEE

Consider whether a project fee or an hourly fee is more appropriate. Generally speaking, a longer project demands a slightly lower hourly rate.

PER-HEAD RATE

A per-head rate is an option if giving a large presentation. This can be structured more than one way. You can charge a certain rate, for example $20 per person, for each attendee. The larger the turnout, the greater your profit. Another option is to charge a flat rate for a guaranteed minimum number of people attending, with an added rate for each additional person over that minimum. You get paid regardless of whether anyone attends. This option presents less risk (6).

VALUE OF THE SERVICE TO THE CLIENT

If the services you are to provide are part of a larger project, and it is necessary for the completion of the project, the practitioner is in a position to demand a high rate.

PRIORITY WORK

If one client wants work done immediately, you may have to put other projects on hold or cancel patients or other billable projects, and this will cost you. You may wish to pass that cost onto the client who requests the priority work.

COMPANY VARIABLES

The size, financial status, and type of company may have an effect on what companies are willing to pay. However, it is important to realize that it is not your job to give your services away to struggling companies.

Mistakes to Avoid

You may see from the above criteria that setting fees is no easy task. In private practice counseling, you will have a set fee schedule. It should now be apparent, however, that a lot of thought must go into the process of setting fees for other contract work.

Never feel like you must immediately state your fee to potential clients. Ask appropriate questions regarding the job—where, what, when, how many, how long, and so on—and tell them you will get back to them. Ask them how soon they need to know, get back to them in a timely manner, but don't let them push you into a fee you will regret.

Remember that once you win the job based on a given fee, you cannot go back with a "whoops, I miscalculated my fees." Therefore, it is always best to overestimate or cushion your fee a bit. Try to start with a high bid for your services and negotiate from that point. Often, you'll be pleasantly surprised that the client will agree to your fees. This strategy will allow for any unforeseeable glitches and will protect you from a potential costly mistake (3).

Most importantly, *do not undersell yourself!* You should ensure that you are getting appropriate compensation for your services, consistent with what your clients are willing to pay. Make sure that the fees that you charge are consistent with the value of your services.

Accounting and Record Keeping

Setting Up Effective Policies and Procedures

It is important that you institute your accounting and other administrative policies before opening your doors. Initially, if you are starting your business on a small scale, you may feel you can just "wing it." This is not recommended. You need to be able to have policies in writing and systems in place. Let's begin with simple record keeping.

Where will you maintain a list of your patients' names, addresses, phone numbers, and other crucial information? Contracts, leases and other legal papers, employee paperwork (if applicable), and licenses all must be kept available as well. Even if some of these items are kept electronically, it is strongly recommended that you keep a hard copy in your filing system (7).

All successful businesses have good bookkeeping and record keeping systems in place. It is imperative to keep detailed records for the following reasons:

- *To monitor and track the performance of your business.* To understand which expenses are necessary and which can be cut, you must constantly monitor your business. Ultimately, this will tell you whether you are making money and assist you in making sound business decisions.

- *To determine your salary.* To know how much to pay yourself, you must know how much you have. It is as simple as that!
- *To track tax obligations.* If you maintain up-to-date, accurate financial records, it is much easier to gather accurate data for filing taxes and other returns or paying quarterly taxes. It will also decrease your accounting bills if you present these detailed records to your accountant when it comes time to preparing your tax returns.
- *To obtain a loan from the bank.* If you want to borrow money, banks request very detailed financial records (7).

Many software packages are available to make detailed record keeping quite simple for small businesses. However, regardless of the computer software program, you still need to enter the data. Information that needs to be entered includes the cash receipts (the money coming in) and the cash disbursements (the money going out).

Each transaction should be recorded and assigned to a category, such as office supplies, rent, postage, etc. If each transaction is accurately recorded, the cash balance on the software package will equal the cash balance in your company checking account. This is known as a balanced set of books. Obviously, this is desirable.

Make sure you save supporting paperwork for your income and expenses. These items may include bank deposit slips, copies of checks, credit card receipts, cancelled checks, bank account statements, invoices, and receipts for out-of-pocket expenses. This material is particularly important should you ever be audited.

To keep your finances straight, you will need to set up your system as if you have two separate businesses. One will manage your accounts receivable and allow you to send invoices out to patients who owe you money. The other will record your income and expenses. That information will be used to file your income taxes and to determine your profits.

Choosing Accounting Software

All the necessary accounting and bookkeeping functions can be performed by software programs. There are many programs available on the market. Choosing the right system for your company is very important. You may want to speak with other business owners who have similar businesses. Also, ask the advice of your accountant.

To help you narrow your choice, consider what functions you want the system to perform. For example, you may want software that provides

---

BOX 4.4

FACTORS TO CONSIDER WHEN CHOOSING ACCOUNTING SOFTWARE

Do you

- Have inventory?

- Need payroll—have employees?

- Want to write checks?

- Want to do bookkeeping for taxes?

- Sell products over the Internet?

- Have international business needs?

- Need to send invoices?

- Need to fax or e-mail invoices?

- Want online banking access?

- Need customized reports?

Source: Data are from Tyson E, Schell J. *Small Business for Dummies.* 2nd ed. New York, NY: John Wiley and Sons Publishing; 2003. and Marshall L. How to choose the right accounting software for your company. Available at: http://www.issi1.com/choose1.html.

---

profit-and-loss statements, writes checks, and sends monthly bills. Box 4.4 lists criteria you may want to consider before purchasing accounting software for your business (8,9). Again, your accountant can certainly advise you. You can also check the Internet for additional resources.

Reimbursement for Services

Many dietetics professionals believe that reimbursement will make or break their practice. This is not necessarily the case. Some dietetics professionals do not accept insurance coverage at all. This also may be a growing trend in medical practices (10). Physicians in some major metropolitan areas are opting out of insurance plans and seeing patients on a fee-for-service basis. They feel they cannot practice medicine with the financial and procedural restrictions placed on them by the insurance companies. This is not a realistic option for many private practice dietitians, however. They find it necessary to accept insurance in order to be successful in private practice.

An important fact to keep in mind is that all health care professionals are competing for the same shrinking reimbursement dollars. Many consumers report that they have to fight for coverage beyond the basic realm of service, such as bone scans, mammograms, and mental health services.

This does not mean, however, that you should throw in the towel. Some dietitians claim that lack of reimbursement has kept them from being successful in their private practices. They are giving up too easily! Dietitians *are* being reimbursed for medical nutrition therapy (MNT).

Information Resources

Private practitioners should stay current with all the reimbursement issues. The information is constantly changing. Fortunately, staying current is made easy through the resources available through ADA. Resources that can help you stay informed include the following:

- The Quality Outcomes and Coverage Team at ADA—members of the team are extremely helpful and available if you have specific questions.
- Your state dietetic association reimbursement representative. He/she should be available to assist you with local issues.
- Your dietetic practice group (DPG) reimbursement chair. He/she should be able to assist you with issues specific to your practice setting.
- ADA's annual Public Policy Workshop held every March in Washington, DC. Attending this meeting allows you to receive the latest information on policy as well as the opportunity to take a trip to Capitol Hill and lobby your representatives.
- Reimbursement manuals and/or materials published by some DPGs. Some sell their resources; others provide them as a free service to their members. Consult the individual DPG Web sites for a listing of materials. You can link to DPG sites through the ADA Web site (http://www.eatright.org).
- Your local library. This is a good place to research business-related information, reimbursement, and policy issues.

Third-Party Payers

Once you have a system in place for staying current, which is crucial if you plan to accept reimbursement, it is important to understand some basic principles. Identifying the types of insurance carriers, referred to as "third-party payers," is the next step in becoming well-versed in the reimbursement arena. At this point, you may want to refer to the glossary in Box 4.5, which defines many terms important in the discussion of reimbursement.

There are different types of third-party payers. The climate in the health care market is changing on a daily basis. Here are some of the more common types of insurance carriers.

BOX 4.5
GLOSSARY OF TERMS

Accept Assignment   A health care provider who participates with an insurance plan. The health care provider agrees to accept the fees specified by the insurance carriers and cannot collect additional fees for the service. In some cases, depending on the specific health plan, the patient pays a portion of the visit.

Beneficiary   Any person who receives insurance benefits from an insurance plan.

CMS 1500   The form that health care providers use to submit Medicare and other insurance claims.

Complementary and Alternative Network (CAM) or Complementary Network (CN)
Networks of practitioners that include services of different practitioners, such as massage therapists, nutritionists/registered dietitians, and chiropractors, who are considered nontraditional. Firms sell both benefit and access services to insurance companies and employer groups, to supplement existing services included in these groups' health benefits plans.

Co-payment   In some health plans, the amount a patient pays for each medical service, like a doctor visit. A co-payment is usually a set amount the patient pays for a service. For example, $5 or $10 for a doctor visit.

CPT (Current Procedural Terminology)   Procedural codes for physicians and other health care professionals, developed by the American Medical Association. Dietetics professionals have specific procedural codes.

Fee for service or Self-Pay   A health care provider provides services to an individual without submitting an insurance claim. The health care provider takes payment for services at the time of the visit.

Health Maintenance Organization (HMO)   A type of health insurance plan that delivers previously determined comprehensive services to its policy holders for a prepaid sum and contracts with or employs health care providers to deliver service.

ICD-9-CM (International Classification of Diseases, 9th edition)   Codes determined by the treating or primary care physician to classify all diagnostic and surgical procedures.

Medicare   The federal health insurance program for people 65 years of age or older, certain younger people with disabilities, and people with End-Stage Renal Disease (those with permanent kidney failure who need regular dialysis or a kidney transplant).

PIN   Acronym for Provider Identification Number. Before billing Medicare, a health care provider must apply for and receive a PIN.

Preferred Provider Organization (PPO)   A health care delivery system that contracts with providers and health care organizations to provide services at discounted fees to members.

Point of Service Organization (POS)   A health plan that offers its members the option of receiving services from participating or nonparticipating providers. Generally, coverage is reduced for services by nonparticipating providers.

Superbill   A preprinted form that itemizes and describes all services and fees. The client can submit directly to the health care insurer.

Sources: Adapted from Hodorowicz M. *Money Matters in Medical Nutrition Therapy Increasing Reimbursement Success in All Practice Settings: The Complete Guide,* 3rd edition (self-published; 2003), with permission of the author, Mary Ann Hodorowicz, MBA, RD, CDE, and from American Dietetic Association. Glossary of Terms. Available at http://www.eatright.org/member/policyinitiatives/83_glossary.cfm. Accessed March 1, 2004. Copyright © American Dietetic Association.

MANAGED CARE ORGANIZATIONS

Managed care organizations—health maintenance organizations (HMOs), preferred provider organizations (PPOs), and point of service organizations (POSs)—require a dietetics professional to be enrolled as a provider in order to be reimbursed for providing medical nutrition therapy or other nutrition services. Usually they also require some form of preauthorization for coverage. They may limit the number of visits annually or for the life of the beneficiary. If you are interested in becoming a provider for managed care organizations, contact provider relations and request an application. In some cases, you may be asked to put your request for an application in writing and even enclose a resume or curriculum vitae. Fill out the required paperwork and send in the necessary supporting documentation. Often they will request a copy of your license (if applicable in your state) and malpractice insurance. The more plans you join, the greater potential for reimbursement (11).

COMMERCIAL PLANS

The dietetics professional may also obtain reimbursement from commercial plans. There are so many commercial plans it is difficult to track them. Note that commercial plans vary from state to state. Even within the same company, the benefits vary from plan to plan. The reimbursement representative from your state dietetic association or your DPG can probably assist you with information on the various plans in your area. Some plans require dietetics professionals to be providers in the same way that managed care organizations do. Others, however, consider each practitioner claim on a case-by-case basis.

COMPLEMENTARY AND ALTERNATIVE MEDICINE NETWORKS

Another option is for the dietetics professional to join networks. These are often referred to as Complementary and Alternative Medicine (CAM) programs or Complementary Networks (CNs). Being a member of a CAM network differs from being a provider. Upon joining the network, the dietetics professional agrees to provide his/her services at a discounted rate to members of that particular plan. In this type of arrangement offered through the CN, the member pays for the service. For example, CareFirst BlueCross BlueShield of Maryland allows patients who have not been diagnosed with an illness requiring nutrition counseling, or who cannot get preauthorization for coverage, to see a dietitian at a discounted rate (12). CNs may also offer benefit CAM services where the employer or insurance pays for the service.

American Specialty Health Networks (ASHN) is a company that has put together a network of dietitians to provide services to members of health plans and employer groups in all 50 states. The ASHN programs offer both discount and benefit plans. With benefit plans, the member pays the dietitian a co-payment (usually between $10 and $20) and the dietitian submits a claim form to ASHN for the contracted reimbursement rate. ASHN reimburses the dietitian for the service. With discount plans, the dietitian provides his/her services to members of the plan at a contracted upon discounted rate.

The ASHN network is unique in that the program is managed by registered dietitians. Treatment plans and credentialing review is all done by the registered dietitian. The program also features online transaction services, so claims are paid quickly and on time. There is no cost to join this network. Its members (more than 65 million in the United States) have access to their programs, and the network has a relationship with more than 150 health plans. Benefits to the dietitian in private practice include a free referral service and the ability to become a provider with several different health plans in one geographical location, all with just one application.

CAM networks are actively pursuing and/or even paying dietetics professionals to join them. Before you join, it is important to determine whether the reimbursement arrangements are a viable option for your practice.

While joining this type of network can potentially increase your referral base, consider the downside. As a member of these networks, you may need to provide deeply discounted fees to members. Some networks are offering set fees that do not differ by geographic region. If you practice in a city where the cost of doing business is high, it may not be worth your time to join. Also, joining these networks may force you to be associated with other practitioners you may not feel are qualified to participate in the CAM network (13). For a complete discussion of the pros and cons of joining CAM networks, refer to reference 14.

MEDICARE

Registered dietitians and other qualifying nutrition professionals are eligible for providing MNT to Medicare beneficiaries. Effective January 1, 2002, patients with diabetes, nondialysis kidney disease, and postkidney transplants can receive the benefit.

The Centers for Medicare and Medicaid Services (CMS) is the government agency that establishes the guidelines and regulations. RDs who want to become Medicare providers must meet specific criteria. The following are some of the RDs' options.

- *Enroll.* Practitioners who meet the provider qualifications can enroll at any time to become a Medicare provider. They must complete and submit CMS Form 855 I (Application for Individual Health Care Practitioners) to their local Medicare carrier. Other enrollment forms may also be required.
- *Do not enroll.* Practitioners who choose not to enroll are not able to provide MNT services to qualifying Medicare beneficiaries unless they opt-out of Medicare Part B. Practitioners cannot provide MNT to any beneficiary with diabetes, nondialysis kidney disease, or post–kidney transplant. They must refer those patients to another registered dietitian who is an enrolled Medicare provider.
- *Opt-out.* In this instance, the practitioner chooses to enter into a private contract with each qualifying Medicare beneficiary in order to provide MNT services. The private contract created for each beneficiary requires very specific requirements, as defined by CMS. The opt-out period is 2 years (14).

For more details on Medicare or policies for opting out, refer to the members-only section of ADA's Web site (http://www.eatright.org/Member/PolicyInitiatives/83_6319.cfm).

If practitioners decide to become Medicare providers, they cannot limit the volume of Medicare patients they see. Some practitioners simply feel they cannot afford to run their businesses on the assigned hourly rates.

Each practice situation is unique and requires careful consideration. Finding the right payer mix that works for your practice will be discussed in greater detail later in this chapter, in the section Accepting Reimbursement.

There are entire manuals devoted to discussing the nuances of Medicare MNT and reimbursement. Chapter 9 lists a number of resources for the dietetics professional who wants to learn more. You could spend an entire day on the ADA Web site (http://www.eatright.org), looking at all the relevant references. This section is in no way comprehensive. Rather, we have highlighted and provided this information as a starting point to learn about reimbursement.

Accepting Reimbursement

Should you decide that accepting reimbursement makes sense for your practice, there are certain administrative tasks you should attend to before the patient's first visit. At the time the appointment is made, obtain the patient's insurance information, making sure a referral will be in place by the time of the appointment, if required. Also, try to find out the reason for the visit, and ask the client to bring a referral including diagnosis information from the physician or physician's office. This is a good time to inform the patient that if MNT is not reimbursed, he/she will be responsible for payment. Patients need to understand that health insurance does not guarantee that all fees and cash will be paid by the insurer. This will allow you to determine coverage before the first visit. If you determine MNT is not covered, you should inform the patient (1). You may need to discuss the advantages and health cost savings they will achieve by receiving nutrition services. Some patients may change their mind about coming to see you based on their financial situation.

After dealing with insurance companies for a while, this task will not be quite as daunting. You will begin to get a feel for the insurance carriers in your area who reimburse for nutrition services. You will have their numbers in your speed dial, and you will streamline your process.

The plans with which RDs contract to provide MNT may have other requirements that affect your practice. For example, Medicare and many private insurance plans require the use of protocols. When furnishing the Medicare MNT benefit, the final regulations state: "RDs and nutritionists would use nationally recognized protocols, such as those developed by the ADA." The guides, titled *Medical Nutrition Therapy (MNT) Evidence-Based Guides for Practice,* are available on CD-ROM from the ADA (15).

[handwritten margin note:] or have it faxed over.

Tools for Billing

Once you have determined that the insurance carrier will reimburse for your services, you must file a claim. This requires either a Superbill or a CMS 1500 form. Different insurance carriers specify which form they accept. Even if you decide not to accept insurance, you should provide your patient with the necessary forms, so that they may file a claim for reimbursement.

Most insurance carriers accept only a completed CMS 1500 form (see Figure 4.2 on page 88). These forms can be purchased from some office supply stores or medical office supply catalogs or can be downloaded from the Centers for Medicare and Medicaid Services Web site (http://www.cms.hhs.gov/providers/edi/cms1500.pdf). Because they cannot be scanned properly, downloaded CMS 1500 forms are not accepted by all insurance companies. These forms are quite time consuming to fill out and must be properly completed to the specifications of the insurance carrier. Forms that are filled out incorrectly or incompletely will be returned to the provider for completion and resubmission. It may be beneficial to purchase a computer software program that can take care of this administrative task.

The CMS 1500 form has a blank space for the taxpayer identification number. The RD can use his/her Social Security number unless he/she has established a corporation for the practice. If you have established a valid corporation or other separate legally recognized entity, which may protect against identity fraud and personal financial liability, a federal tax identification number must be obtained (1). In addition, Medicare RD providers also include their Medicare Provider Identification Number (PIN) on the CMS 1500 form.

Filing claims electronically is becoming more common. This eliminates the need to mail forms to insurance carriers. Instead, claims are sent via the Internet. Some insurance carriers enable you to submit your claims on their Web sites or give their contracted providers the necessary software to enable them to file claims electronically. The software may have a fee associated with it, so make sure to check first. It is critical that you abide by the Health Insurance Portability and Accountability Act (refer to Chapter 3) when filing electronic claims.

There are many companies and organizations that provide medical billing products, educational materials for practitioners, and other resources. Box 4.6 (see page 89) lists some companies and organizations that provide medical billing products. Check the telephone book under "insurance claim processing services" or "medical billing," search the Internet, or contact your local insurance carriers for additional resources (16). For the dietetics professional who plans to handle a multitude of insurance claims, using one of these companies to handle insurance billing could be a wise investment.

FIGURE 4.2

Sample CMS 1500 form.

PLEASE
DO NOT
STAPLE
IN THIS
AREA

CARRIER

PICA **HEALTH INSURANCE CLAIM FORM** PICA

1. MEDICARE (Medicare #) MEDICAID (Medicaid #) CHAMPUS (Sponsor's SSN) CHAMPVA (VA File #) GROUP HEALTH PLAN (SSN or ID) FECA BLK LUNG (SSN) OTHER (ID)

1a. INSURED'S I.D. NUMBER (FOR PROGRAM IN ITEM 1)

2. PATIENT'S NAME (Last Name, First Name, Middle Initial)

3. PATIENT'S BIRTH DATE MM DD YY SEX M F

4. INSURED'S NAME (Last Name, First Name, Middle Initial)

5. PATIENT'S ADDRESS (No., Street)

6. PATIENT RELATIONSHIP TO INSURED Self Spouse Child Other

7. INSURED'S ADDRESS (No., Street)

CITY STATE

8. PATIENT STATUS Single Married Other

CITY STATE

ZIP CODE TELEPHONE (Include Area Code) ( )

Employed Full-Time Student Part-Time Student

ZIP CODE TELEPHONE (INCLUDE AREA CODE) ( )

9. OTHER INSURED'S NAME (Last Name, First Name, Middle Initial)

10. IS PATIENT'S CONDITION RELATED TO:

11. INSURED'S POLICY GROUP OR FECA NUMBER

a. OTHER INSURED'S POLICY OR GROUP NUMBER

a. EMPLOYMENT? (CURRENT OR PREVIOUS) YES NO

a. INSURED'S DATE OF BIRTH MM DD YY SEX M F

b. OTHER INSURED'S DATE OF BIRTH MM DD YY SEX M F

b. AUTO ACCIDENT? PLACE (State) YES NO

b. EMPLOYER'S NAME OR SCHOOL NAME

c. EMPLOYER'S NAME OR SCHOOL NAME

c. OTHER ACCIDENT? YES NO

c. INSURANCE PLAN NAME OR PROGRAM NAME

d. INSURANCE PLAN NAME OR PROGRAM NAME

10d. RESERVED FOR LOCAL USE

d. IS THERE ANOTHER HEALTH BENEFIT PLAN? YES NO *If yes,* return to and complete item 9 a-d.

READ BACK OF FORM BEFORE COMPLETING & SIGNING THIS FORM.

12. PATIENT'S OR AUTHORIZED PERSON'S SIGNATURE I authorize the release of any medical or other information necessary to process this claim. I also request payment of government benefits either to myself or to the party who accepts assignment below.

SIGNED DATE

13. INSURED'S OR AUTHORIZED PERSON'S SIGNATURE I authorize payment of medical benefits to the undersigned physician or supplier for services described below.

SIGNED

PATIENT AND INSURED INFORMATION

14. DATE OF CURRENT: MM DD YY ILLNESS (First symptom) OR INJURY (Accident) OR PREGNANCY(LMP)

15. IF PATIENT HAS HAD SAME OR SIMILAR ILLNESS. GIVE FIRST DATE MM DD YY

16. DATES PATIENT UNABLE TO WORK IN CURRENT OCCUPATION FROM MM DD YY TO MM DD YY

17. NAME OF REFERRING PHYSICIAN OR OTHER SOURCE

17a. I.D. NUMBER OF REFERRING PHYSICIAN

18. HOSPITALIZATION DATES RELATED TO CURRENT SERVICES FROM MM DD YY TO MM DD YY

19. RESERVED FOR LOCAL USE

20. OUTSIDE LAB? YES NO $ CHARGES

21. DIAGNOSIS OR NATURE OF ILLNESS OR INJURY. (RELATE ITEMS 1,2,3 OR 4 TO ITEM 24E BY LINE)

1. ___ . ___
2. ___ . ___
3. ___ . ___
4. ___ . ___

22. MEDICAID RESUBMISSION CODE ORIGINAL REF. NO.

23. PRIOR AUTHORIZATION NUMBER

24. A DATE(S) OF SERVICE From MM DD YY To MM DD YY	B Place of Service	C Type of Service	D PROCEDURES, SERVICES, OR SUPPLIES (Explain Unusual Circumstances) CPT/HCPCS MODIFIER	E DIAGNOSIS CODE	F $ CHARGES	G DAYS OR UNITS	H EPSDT Family Plan	I EMG	J COB	K RESERVED FOR LOCAL USE
1										
2										
3										
4										
5										
6										

25. FEDERAL TAX I.D. NUMBER SSN EIN

26. PATIENT'S ACCOUNT NO.

27. ACCEPT ASSIGNMENT? (For govt. claims, see back) YES NO

28. TOTAL CHARGE $

29. AMOUNT PAID $

30. BALANCE DUE $

31. SIGNATURE OF PHYSICIAN OR SUPPLIER INCLUDING DEGREES OR CREDENTIALS (I certify that the statements on the reverse apply to this bill and are made a part thereof.)

SIGNED DATE

32. NAME AND ADDRESS OF FACILITY WHERE SERVICES WERE RENDERED (If other than home or office)

33. PHYSICIAN'S, SUPPLIER'S BILLING NAME, ADDRESS, ZIP CODE & PHONE #

PIN# GRP#

PHYSICIAN OR SUPPLIER INFORMATION

(APPROVED BY AMA COUNCIL ON MEDICAL SERVICE 8/88) ***PLEASE PRINT OR TYPE*** APPROVED OMB-0938-0008 FORM CMS-1500 (12/90), FORM RRB-1500, APPROVED OMB-1215-0055 FORM OWCP-1500, APPROVED OMB-0720-0001 (CHAMPUS)

BOX 4.6
BILLING RESOURCES

Government

Centers for Medicare & Medicaid Services (CMS)
http://cms.hhs.gov/medicare/edi

As part of the Health Insurance Portability and Accountability Act (HIPAA), CMS offers program updates and publication notices through the Electronic Data Interchange (EDI) electronic mailing list. Free Medicare Electronic Media Claim (EMC) software is also available.

Nonprofit

National Electronic Billers Alliance (NEBA)
http://www.nebazone.com

Reportedly the largest medical billing organization in the country, NEBA offers education, information, and software to professional medical billers. NEBA also certifies professional billers as "Health Care Reimbursement Specialists." Their Web site includes news, discussion, and membership information.

American Medical Billing Association (AMBA)
http://www.ambanet.net

AMBA provides networking and some advocacy for small and home-based professional medical billers. Their Web site features software packages and a list of vendors with AMBA's Medical Billing Certification.

Medical Billing Network
http://www.medicalbillingnetwork.com

The Medical Billing Network is a trade association and school for both small and large independent medical billers. They offer several electronic medical billing software products on their Web page.

Web-based

Medicalbillingworld.com
http://www.medicalbillingworld.com/index.html

An online outlet for medical billing books, forms, software, and customer service. Review its entire inventory at the Web site.

Source: Data are from American Dietetic Association. Billing Resources. Available at: http://www.eatright.org/member/policy/initiatives/83_billresource.cfm.

Superbill

The Superbill is a different type of claim form (see Figure 4.3). This bill is more commonly used in a practice where the filing is not done electronically. You may not even be filing claims at all. Rather, they are filled out manually by the dietitian at the end of each visit. The dietitian provides the patient with a Superbill, with the understanding that the insurance company may or may not pay for the counseling. This puts the onus of collecting reimbursement on the patient.

A Superbill must have certain components. Refer to Box 4.7 (see page 92) for a thorough listing. You can create your own Superbill using your computer, or you can purchase camera-ready Superbills.

One component of the Superbill is the ICD-9-CM codes. ICD-9 CM stands for the International Classification of Diseases, 9th revision (6th edition), Clinical Modifications. The ICD-9-CM book is the manual that contains a listing of the diagnoses codes. You can purchase a manual through the American Medical Association (http://www.ama-assn.org) or from the local bookstore. There are also resources on the Internet where you can obtain this information. One such Web site is run by the Stanford University School of Medicine (http://neuro3.stanford.edu/CodeWorrier). Refer to Box 4.8 (see pages 92–93) for a listing of diagnosis codes.

Two more critical notes: First, it is important to obtain a correct diagnosis code(s) from the patient's physician. RDs cannot determine the medical diagnosis; this is not in the RD's scope of practice. Second, if the physician provides the primary diagnosis and diagnosis codes for comorbidity, some health providers may increase coverage.

CPT Codes

CPT Codes, or Physician's Current Procedural Terminology, are the office procedural codes. The 2001 CPT manual contains specific codes for MNT counseling by registered dietitians. The MNT codes are time based. Individual codes are based on 15-minute units and group codes on 30-minute units. They can be billed in multiple units. For example, if the initial MNT is 60 minutes, four units are billed. Refer to Box 4.9 (see page 94) for MNT codes.

FIGURE 4.3

Sample Superbill. Reprinted with permission from Pennsylvania Dietetic Association, © 2002.

MEDICAL NUTRITION THERAPY STATEMENT

SUBSCRIBER'S NAME _____ DATE _____

PATIENT'S NAME _____ PATIENT'S DATE OF BIRTH _____

ADDRESS _____

INSURANCE CO. _____ POLICY NO. _____ GROUP NO. _____

ICD-9 Codes

☐	783.1	Abnormal Weight Gain	☐	558.9	Gastroenteritis	☐	627.2	Menopausal Syndrome
☐	783.2	Abnormal Weight Loss	☐	530.81	Gastroesophageal Reflux	☐	412	Myocardial Infection
☐	285.9	Anemia, Unspecified	☐	271.3	Glucose Intolerance	☐	278.0	Obesity
☐	307.1	Anorexia Nervosa	☐	579.0	Gluten Sensitive Enteropathy	☐	733.00	Osteoporosis
☐	716.90	Arthritis	☐	274.9	Gout	☐	332.0	Parkinsonism
☐	493.90	Asthma	☐	042.0	HIV Infection	☐	533.0	Peptic Ulcer Disease
☐	414.0	Arteriosclerotic Heart			w/ Specified Infections	☐	270.1	PKU
		Disorder (ASHD)	☐	272.2	Hyperlipidemia	☐	564.2	Post Gastrectomy Syndrome
☐	564.1	Bowel, Irritable Syndrome	☐	401.9	Hypertension, Essential	☐	V22.2	Pregnancy, Normal
☐	307.51	Bulimia	☐	242.9	Hyperthyroidism	☐	593.9	Renal Disease
☐	574.20	Cholelithiasis	☐	251.2	Hypoglycemia	☐	780.5	Sleep Apnea
☐	585	Chronic Renal Failure	☐	244.9	Hypothyroidism	☐	556.9	Ulcerative Colitis
☐	749.2	Cleft Palate with Cleft Lip	☐	646.8	Insufficient Weight Gain,	☐	269.2	Vitamin Deficiency
☐	428.0	Congestive Heart Failure			Pregnancy	☐		Other _____
☐	564.0	Constipation	☐	271.3	Lactose Intolerance			
☐	555.9	Crohn's Disease	☐	263.9	Malnutrition			
☐	277.00	Cystic Fibrosis						
☐	722.6	Deg. Disc Disease						
☐	715.90	Deg. Joint Disease						
☐	648.8	Diabetes, Gestational						
☐	250.01	Diabetes, Type 1						
☐	250.00	Diabetes, Type 2						
☐	648.0	Diabetes with Pregnancy						
☐	250.4	Diabetic Nephropathy						
☐	558.9	Diarrhea						
☐	562.11	Diverticulitis						
☐	562.10	Diverticulosis						
☐	787.2	Dysphagia						
☐	307.5	Eating Disorder, Unspecified						
☐	646.1	Excess Weight Gain,						
		Pregnancy						
☐	783.4	Failure to Thrive/						
		Physical Retardation						
☐	693.1	Food Allergy						
☐	535.4	Gastritis						

Services _____

MNT CPT Codes, if applicable

☐ 97802 Initial assessment & intervention, individual, face-to-face

Each unit = 15 minutes _____ Units

☐ 97803 Re-assessment & intervention, individual, face-to-face

Each unit = 15 minutes _____ Units

☐ 97804 Group (2 or more), each 30 minutes _____ Units

Other CPT Code, if applicable

☐ Initial Eval. & Consultation

☐ Follow-Up Consultation _____ Total Charge

☐ Nutr. Assess, Comprehensive _____ Amount Paid

☐ Phone Consultation _____ Balance Due

☐ Instructional Material

☐ Diet Instructions

☐ Other: _____

RD Name _____ RD Signature _____ Date _____

RD # _____ Provider # _____ Phone # _____

Address _____

WHITE - Office Copy   YELLOW - Insurance Copy   PINK - Patient Copy

BOX 4.7

COMPONENTS OF A SUPERBILL

- Provider name
- Provider address
- Provider telephone/fax numbers
- RD number (not required but adds credibility)
- License number (if applicable in your state)
- Tax identification number (TIN) or Social Security number
- Patient name
- Date of service
- Diagnosis code (from International Classification of Diseases, 9th revision [ICD-9-CM])
- Procedural code (Current Procedural Terminology or CPT)
- Fee for service
- Payment
- Balance due
- Provider signature

BOX 4.8

ICD-9-CM CODES COMMONLY USED BY DIETETICS PROFESSIONALS*

783.1	Abnormal weight gain
783.2	Abnormal weight loss
285.9	Anemia, unspecified
307.1	Anorexia nervosa
716.90	Arthritis
493.60	Asthma
414.0	Arteriosclerotic heart disorder (ASHD)
564.1	Bowel, irritable bowel syndrome
307.51	Bulimia
574.20	Cholelithiasis
585	Chronic renal failure
749.2	Cleft palate with cleft lip
428.0	Congestive heart failure
564.0	Constipation
555.9	Crohn's disease
277.0	Cystic fibrosis
722.6	Degenerative disc disease
715.90	Degenerative joint disease

648.8	Diabetes, gestational
250.01	Diabetes, type 1
250.00	Diabetes, type 2
648.0	Diabetes with pregnancy
250.4	Diabetic nephropathy
558.8	Diarrhea
562.11	Diverticulitis
562.10	Diverticulosis
787.2	Dysphagia
307.5	Eating disorder, unspecified
646.1	Excess weight gain, pregnancy
783.4	Failure to thrive/Physical retardation
693.1	Food allergy
535.4	Gastritis
558.9	Gastroenteritis
530.81	Gastroesophageal reflux
271.3	Glucose intolerance
579.0	Gluten-sensitive enteropathy
274.9	Gout
042.0	HIV infection with specified infections
272.2	Hyperlipidemia
401.9	Hypertension, essential
242.9	Hyperthyroidism
251.2	Hypoglycemia
244.9	Hypothyroidism
646.8	Insufficient weight gain, pregnancy
271.3	Lactose intolerance
263.9	Malnutrition
627.2	Menopausal syndrome
412	Myocardial infection
277.0	Obesity
733.00	Osteoporosis
332.0	Parkinsonism
533.0	Peptic ulcer disease
270.1	PKU
564.1	Postgastrectomy syndrome
V22.2	Pregnancy, normal
593.9	Renal disease
780.5	Sleep apnea
556.9	Ulcerative colitis
269.2	Vitamin deficiency

*Always consult International Classification of Diseases, 9th revision (ICD-9-CM) to confirm the accuracy of all codes. ICD-9-CM can be purchased from the American Medical Association (http://www.ama-assn.org); codes are also published on some Web sites.

BOX 4.9

MEDICAL NUTRITION THERAPY (MNT) CODES

97802   MNT, initial assessment and intervention, individual, face-to-face with the patient, each 15 minutes

97803   Reassessment and intervention, individual, face-to-face with the patient, each 15 minutes

97804   Group (2 or more individuals), each 30 minutes

For MNT services on or after January 1, 2003, CMS requires the use of two new MNT codes for billing additional hours of MNT beyond the 3 hours of initial episode of care in the first calendar year and beyond two hours of follow-up episode of care in each subsequent calendar year when the physician determines there is a change in diagnosis or medical condition that makes a change in diet necessary.

G0270   MNT reassessment and subsequent intervention(s) following second referral in same year for change in diagnosis, medical condition, or treatment regimen (including additional house needed for renal disease), individual, face-to-face with the patient, each 15 minutes.

G0271   MNT reassessment and subsequent intervention(s) following second referral in same year for change in diagnosis, medical condition, or treatment regimen (including additional hours needed for renal disease) group (2 or more individuals), each 30 minutes.

Source: Current procedural terminology (CPT) codes, descriptions, and material only are copyright © 2000 American Medical Association. All Rights Reserved.

Reimbursement Policies: What's Right for Your Practice?

Options

With some understanding of reimbursement, your fees established, and your accounting system in place, you are ready to determine which reimbursement policies work best for you. Consider the following options.

FEE FOR SERVICE

The dietetics professional does not participate with any insurance plans. She/he informs patients when they call for an appointment that payment is expected at the time of the visit. The patient will be provided with a Superbill and encouraged to file for reimbursement with their insurance company. Although this may deter some potential patients from scheduling appointments, some RDs argue that individuals who choose to pay for services are more serious about implementing dietary changes.

ACCEPTING ASSIGNMENT

The dietetics professional becomes a provider for managed care organizations, commercial plans, and/or the government, as a Medicare provider. A co-payment is generally collected from the patient at the time of the visit. A claim is then filed with the patient's insurance carrier, or the government for Medicare claims, for reimbursement for services. When you accept assignment, you may be bound by the policies of the various insurance carriers. There may be limits on the number of visits a patient is authorized for, patients may require preauthorization before seeing you, and there may be predetermined reimbursement rates. Although this approach can increase your volume of patients, particularly when you are first getting started, the amount of paperwork required is much greater than in other methods. You must determine eligibility before the patient comes in, file the claim, track which claims have been paid, frequently re-file the claim, and possibly bill the patient if the claim is denied.

COMBINATIONS

This is not an all-or-nothing decision. Many private practitioners use a combination of methods. They have some fee-for-service patients, particularly those patients who have elected to see them for wellness, weight-management issues, or with non-nutrition-related diagnoses. They also have some patients for whom they are filing insurance claims.

Practice Models

For another way to analyze which approach best fits your practice needs, consider the following practice models (17).

MEDICARE CLIENTS ONLY

It is possible to base your practice solely on Medicare clients. The beneficiaries do require a physician referral. If you have a few good referral sources, you can maintain a steady stream of clients. Medicare beneficiaries can receive three hours of coverage in the first three years and two hours in subsequent years, so you will need a constant source of new referrals. Becoming a Medicare provider requires having the necessary systems in place to comply with regulations. Some potential pitfalls of a Medicare-based practice include the possibility that the reimbursement rate may not meet your salary expectations or adequately cover your business expenses, administrative duties are likely to increase, and your client base will be limited to the diseases and conditions Medicare covers, such as diabetes and renal disease.

PAYER MIX, MEDICARE OPT-OUT

The dietetics professional sees clients and Medicare beneficiaries who pay out-of-pocket for service. He/she is also a provider for one or more insurance plans that directly reimburse the dietetics professional. He/she is not a provider of Medicare MNT and is only able to provide MNT to Medicare beneficiaries through the government's opting out regulations. Potentially, this scenario may bring higher payment rates. It also provides a more varied client population. Consider the downsides of this model. Opting out of Medicare may reduce your referrals and you may have to increase your marketing efforts to compensate. Also, there may be ramifications of opting out of Medicare. One such ramification is that the opt-out period is for two years, so opting out could potentially impact the dietetics professional's future employment opportunities (18).

PAYER BLEND INCLUDING MEDICARE

This model encompasses all scenarios. The dietetics professional is a provider for Medicare, for private insurance plans, and accepts self-pay patients. This model may offer a larger volume of clients and a greater income. The higher reimbursement rates received from private insurance and self-pay clients can offset the Medicare rates. Conversely, the Medicare clients provide steady referrals. A potential pitfall of this model is that it requires a great amount of organization to track numerous claims and to manage contracts and billing.

SELF-PAY CLIENTS ONLY

Sometimes referred to as fee for service, this model is one in which the dietetics professional is not a provider for Medicare or private insurance plans. This model does have the potential for higher payment rates and requires much less administrative work for the dietetics professional. With less time spent on administrative duties, more time can be spent seeing patients and billing for that time. The dietetics professional can become highly specialized in this case, and patients will seek her/him for the particular specialty niche. For example, an eating disorders, weight management, or women's health specialist may wish to build a fee-for-service practice. Along with the previously mentioned pitfalls associated with opting out of Medicare, not becoming a provider for even private insurance companies has the potential to greatly reduce your client base and income. You also must expend extra time and effort in marketing your services.

Box 4.10 provides a summary of the pros and cons of the practice models discussed in this chapter.

Accounting and Reimbursement Issues to Consider

If you are seeing both private pay and insurance patients, it is important to have a system for tracking outstanding insurance claims while keeping your private billing separate (if you are not billing insurance carriers electronically). You may be able to suppress statements on those accounts that are waiting for insurance reimbursement.

As already mentioned in Chapter 3, regardless of which route you decide to take, each new patient needs to read and sign your reimbursement

---

BOX 4.10

SELECTING A DIETETICS PRACTICE MODEL

Model 1: Medicare Clients

Pros:

• Stable and predictable

• Potential for large number of clientele

• Minimal marketing

• Opportunity for follow-up

• Good systems development

• Recognition as a Medicare provider

(continues)

BOX 4.10 (continued)

Cons:

- Reimbursement rate may not meet salary requirements
- Administrative duties
- Medicare clients limited to diabetes and renal

Model 2: Private Pay, Third Party Payers, and Opting Out of Medicare

Pros:

- Potential for higher payment rate
- Broader range of clients' payment rate
- Provider status with private plans

Cons:

- Requires marketing and negotiating skills
- May be less stable
- May reduce referrals
- Ramifications of opting out of Medicare

Model 3: Medicare and Third Party Payers, Plus Self-Pay Clients

Pros:

- Variety and professional satisfaction
- Success with Medicare generates non-Medicare referrals
- Maintains client flow
- Builds skills and confidence with billing and negotiating systems
- Benefit from economies of scale as a result of time and experience

Cons:

- Requires up-front work to stay organized and efficient with time
- Management of contracts and billing

Model 4: Self-Pay Clients

Pros:

- Potential for higher payment rate
- Less administrative work
- Frequently used with highly specialized practices
- Dietetics professional can establish a wellness-based practice

Cons:

- Requires constant creative marketing
- May be less stable
- May reduce referrals

Source: Adapted with permission from *MNT Medicare Provider,* January 2004, p.2. Copyright © 2004 American Dietetic Association.

policies. This document must clearly state your policies, so that the patient understands that they are ultimately responsible for the bill should their insurance not pay.

It is important to note that reimbursement is being provided for MNT. Registered dietitians who file insurance claims are regularly being reimbursed by insurance carriers for MNT. As a result, many have thriving nutrition practices as providers for multiple insurance carriers. Patients who file for themselves are also being reimbursed for MNT. If provided with an accurately completed Superbill, they are encouraged to file a claim with their insurance carrier. If the initial claim is denied, encourage them to resubmit the claim. Teach patients to advocate for themselves, so that they can receive reimbursement.

Professional Example: One Dietitian's Reimbursement Policies

Ann Silver, MS, RD, CDE, CDN, has a private practice with offices in West Hampton Beach and East Hampton, New York. She is a provider for numerous insurance carriers, including Medicare. Therefore, most of her patients pay only a co-pay to see her. Ann then files a claim with the patient's insurance company for reimbursement based on a set fee schedule per CPT code.

All the insurance billing for Ms. Silver's practice is done by electronic billing through a company called ProxyMed. This service, furnished to providers with the insurance carriers she participates with, generates a claim for each patient encounter.

Ann has two forms that she uses in her private practice. They assist her in tracking the insurance claims. Each new patient fills out a New Patient Form (Figure 4.4 on page 101). Additionally, she obtains the patient's insurance information—insurance company, ID number, co-pay, etc.—and makes a copy of their insurance card. On the bottom of that form is a section "for office use only." This becomes a tracking section for Ann to determine when reimbursement, insurance, and self-pay has been posted to the billing company and when she has received it.

Another important tool Ms. Silver uses in her practice is her Daily Services Rendered Form (Figure 4.5; see page 102). At the end of each day she uses this form to summarize her daily billings. She is able to determine which patients she saw each day and list all their pertinent insurance information, their diagnosis, and CPT code, with the number of units billed, the fee for service, co-pay remitted, and their next appointment. This form also enables Ann to monitor reimbursement and daily production.

Ann makes sure to determine whether each patient is responsible for a co-payment by checking the insurance card at the first visit. She is vigilant about collecting the co-pay at each visit. For those patients who come to see her without insurance coverage (fee for service), Ann specifies that payment is due when services are rendered. This way she limits her accounts receivable to pending insurance claims.

Money Management: A Summary

There are many business decisions to make before you begin your new venture. If making all these decisions seems overwhelming, consider seeking the advice of professionals, such as accountants, business advisors, or other dietetics professionals. Some private practitioners are available to budding entrepreneurs on a consulting basis. Remember, they too must be paid for their professional services. Budget accordingly, and seek professional advice when necessary. Additionally, keep the following points in mind:

- It is imperative to set office policies before you see patients. All patients should be informed of your policies when they schedule their first appointment and in writing at the time of their first visit.
- Some dietetics professionals are strictly fee for service. They inform the patient that payment is due at the time of the visit. The patient files an insurance claim for self-reimbursement.
- You must also have policies in place for billing, collecting past due accounts, returned checks, cancellations, and no-show appointments.
- When setting fees, factor in your desired salary, cost to replace lost benefits, business and office expenses, and your salable time.
- Closely monitoring your finances is extremely important to assist you in determining the viability of your new company. Choosing the right accounting software will help.
- RDs across the United States are being reimbursed for MNT by commercial insurance plans, managed care organizations, complementary and alternative medicine networks, and Medicare.

FIGURE 4.4

New patient registration form.

NEW PATIENT REGISTRATION

Patient's Name:_____ Date:_____

Mailing Address: _____

City: _____ State: _____ Zip Code: _____

Home Phone: _____ Work Phone: _____ E-mail: _____

Date of Birth: _____ Age: _____ Social Security Number: _____

Patient's Occupation: _____ Employer: _____

Primary Insurance Company:_____

     Insurance ID#:_____ Co-pay $:_____

Primary Insured's Name: _____Primary Insured's Date of Birth:_____
(Insured's name is not necessarily the patient's name, but the family member who has the insurance.)

Insured's Employer: _____

Secondary Insurance Company: _____

Insurance ID #: _____

Secondary Insured's Name: _____ Secondary Insured's Date of Birth: _____
(Insured's name is not necessarily the patient's name, but the family member who has the insurance.)

Primary Physician's Name: _____Physician's Phone: _____

Physician's Address: _____

Referring Physician's Name: _____Physician's Phone: _____

FOR OFFICE USE

DOS	REFFERAL #	ICD	CPT/UNITS	FEE	POSTED	COPAY	PAYMENT AMT/DATE

FIGURE 4.5

Form for tracking daily services rendered.

Date of service: _____

Patient name	Ins.	ID#	Referral #	DOB	CPT/units	ICD-9 codes	Fee	Posted	Co-pay	Paid	Other info	Next appt

- The RD's options for involvement in enrollment in the Medicare MNT benefit include enrolling to become a provider, choosing not to enroll, or opting out.
- The RD should use a Superbill if method of payment is fee for service. If the RD is filing insurance claims, a CMS 1500 form should be used. Using proper MNT and ICD-9 codes are required for successful claims processing.

References

1. Liskov T. Putting together the pieces on reimbursement—getting started in private practice. *Dietitian's Edge.* May-June 2001:44–48.
2. Georgia B. The price is tight . . . isn't it? (industry trend or event). *Home Office Computing.* June 1999. Available at: http://findarticles.com/cf_0/ml1563/6_17/63502624/print.html. Accessed November 7, 2003.
3. Duester K. Building your business—setting your fees: a cost-based approach. *J Am Diet Assoc.* 1997:97(suppl):S129–S130.
4. Axelrod M. The consulting process: setting fees. Available at: http://www.thenewgame.com/axelrodlearning/consultingprocess.html. Accessed November 6, 2003.
5. Croasdale M. The price is right: when patients want to haggle. *Am Med News.* May 6, 2002. Available at: http://www.ama-assn.org/amednews/2002/05/06/bisa0506.htm. Accessed March 8, 2004.
6. King K. *The Entrepreneurial Nutritionist.* Lake Dallas, Tex: Helm Publishing; 2002.
7. Mintzer R. *The Everything to Start Your Own Business Book.* Avon, Mass: Adams Media Corporation; 2002.
8. Tyson E, Schell J. *Small Business for Dummies.* 2nd ed. New York, NY: John Wiley and Sons Publishing; 2003.
9. Marshall L. How to choose the right accounting software for your company. Available at: http://www.issi1.com/choose1.html. Accessed December 4, 2003.
10. Borbely M. This may hurt; some doctors are spurning managed care, giving more time—and a bigger bill—to their patients. *Washington Post.* October 30, 2001:HE01.
11. Larson E. Understanding MNT coding and reimbursement. [American Dietetic Association Web site]. Available at: http://www.eatright.org/member/83_resources.cfm. Accessed December 6, 2003.
12. Fiske H. Insurance and nutrition counseling. *Today's Dietitian.* 2003;6:25–27.
13. American Dietetic Association Health Care Financing and Quality Management Team. *Medicare MNT Benefit Provider Information.* Chicago, Ill: American Dietetic Association; 2002.
14. Albarado M. Understanding and negotiating access contracts with insurers and complementary networks. *J Am Diet Assoc.* 2002;102:187–189.

15. Shanklin C. Evidence-based practice: practice based evidence, right? *ADA Times.* 2003;1:1–3.

16. American Dietetic Association. Billing Resources. Available at: http://www.eatright.org/member/policy/initiatives/83_billresource.cfm. Accessed December 8, 2003.

17. Finding the practice model that fits your business needs. *The Medicare MNT Provider.* 2004;2:1–3.

18. Infante M, Michael P, Pritchett E. Opting out of Medicare: a serious business decision. *J Am Diet Assoc.* 2002;102:1061–1062.

Chapter 5

Marketing

You may be on the cutting edge of diabetes management, have written a bestseller, or have the greatest success rate with helping breastfeeding mothers, but if no one knows about you, then your business or product fails. Success in business is all about marketing. Marketing separates you from your competition. Good marketing translates into a successful business.

To market effectively, you must build a plan around the 4 Ps of marketing: *Product, Place, Price,* and *Promotion.* These topics can be systematically addressed by creating a marketing plan. The marketing plan is different from the business plan addressed in Chapter 2. A business plan is your blueprint for getting your business to the customer. Your marketing plan is a strategic plan to get your name and your business to the consumer. It isn't theoretical; it's a practical plan of action (1–4).

Many small businesses may develop a business plan but stumble through the marketing process. Reasons offered for ignoring marketing plans include insufficient cash, lack of knowledge, and its being of low priority. To successfully market your services, your plan will define the following:

- Your target market
- The service or product you are selling
- Tools you will use to ensure that your product reaches the market

It is as basic as that. Don't get too bogged down with the fine points. Whether you are marketing your private practice or a new nutrition product, you need to develop a plan that will be revised, refined, and reformulated as your business develops.

Your Target Market

Who needs your services? Although those in the nutrition profession might feel that everyone can benefit from seeing a dietitian, marketing your services requires you to be a bit more specific and objective. To identify your target market, you will need to learn characteristics of the population you wish to reach, your competition, and how your services are being priced in the marketplace. You must also find out about trends in the marketplace and answer how (or if) your target market is presently having their needs met.

Your research will help you learn about the demographics of the population you wish to reach. What is their age group? What is their socioeconomic profile? Where are they now turning for the service you hope to offer them? This is the research that will help you to conclude where your practice or service is the most needed or will be most likely to succeed.

Conducting an analysis of the marketplace will help you to identify what services are being provided and what is missing. If you are in an area where there are already some other dietitians practicing, assess what needs are not being met. This allows you to position your practice advantageously.

Thorough marketing research should reveal information about your competition. Your competitors will include other dietetics professionals, commercial programs, chiropractors, outpatient departments of local hospitals, and health food stores, to name a few. Your goal in assessing the competition is to determine how your services will meet a client's needs in a way that the competition does not.

Analyze the competition by assessing their strengths and weakness. Compare them to your own. To create uniqueness, ask yourself what is special about your services? This might focus on practical questions such as the following:

- Is your office location accessible by public transportation?
- Do you accept credit cards?
- Do you work evenings or Saturdays?

For further assistance in this assessment, see Box 5.1 (5).

Tools for obtaining information about your competition range from constructing a formal survey that is mailed to your identified audience to something as simple as picking up the telephone and calling commercial programs, local hospitals, wellness centers, and other dietetics professionals in private practice.

Many dietetics professionals view their competition as the enemy. This is a shortsighted analysis. In fact, other dietitians in private practice can be your greatest referral source, if you market yourself properly. A careful analysis of your own strengths and weaknesses will allow you to refer to other dietetics professionals when you cannot meet a patient's needs. This not only allows you to assist a patient, but it also may result in reciprocal referrals from other dietetics professionals. Referrals result in a win-win relationship.

To find out which services are needed most or how your desired service is doing in the marketplace, you need to track consumer trends. Read

BOX 5.1
EVALUATING THE COMPETITION

1. Competitor's name: _____

2. Location: _____

    Accessible by public transportation? _____

3. Days and hours of business: _____

4. Years in business: _____

5. Specialist or generalist: _____

6. If specialist, what is the specialty? _____

7. Price for services: _____

8. Methods of payment accepted:

    Managed care_____

    Fee for service_____

    Credit cards_____

    Strengths of competitor (the strengths become your strengths)_____

    Weaknesses (looking at the weaknesses of the competition can help you find ways of being unique and benefiting the consumer) _____

Source: Adapted with permission from Pinson L, Jinnett J. *Steps to Small Business Start-Up. Everything You Need to Know to Turn Your Idea into a Successful Business.* Chicago, Ill: Dearborn; 2000:242. Copyright © 2000 Dearborn Trade Publishing.

annual reports from trade organizations, professional publications, and government publications. Immediate information on trends is available just by reading newspapers and magazines. They can provide insight into what readers think is hot, what foods they are purchasing, present diet fads, or where people are exercising. Although you don't need to be a part of every diet trend, you do need to be aware of the trends in order to speak convincingly to your clients. It is not necessary to be the first, just the best. Box 5.2 provides additional guidance for determining trends.

Formal marketing research can be daunting and quite costly, especially for the new dietetics professional just getting started in practice. Think outside the box to get the information you need, without spending your entire marketing budget. Research doesn't have to be obtained by professionally developed questionnaires or sophisticated market surveys. To keep expenses down and methods manageable, you can use some creative resources that are readily available to you.

BOX 5.2
TRACKING FOOD AND NUTRITION TRENDS

- ADA's Daily News Report: A daily e-mail newsletter that informs ADA members of news relating to food, nutrition, and health. Sign up at the ADA Web site (http://www.eatright.org).

- Food Marketing Institute Report: This annual research study tracks consumer behavior and attitudes on a wide range of issues that are important to understanding the grocery shopper. Topics include spending patterns, satisfaction ratings, importance of products and services, types of stores shopped, nutrition and food safety concerns. More information can be found at the Food Marketing Institute's Web site (http://www.FMI.org).

- Marketresearch.com: A Web site that compiles and sells market research reports by industry, market research publisher, and geographic area. More information can be found at the Web site (http://www.marketresearch.com).

- Trendwatching.com: A Web site that focuses on consumer insights and behavioral trends, and the hands-on marketing/business opportunities they present. Provides a free monthly newsletter. More information can be found at the Web site (http://www.trendwatching.com).

- Consumer Trends Forum International: CTFI is a nonprofit organization that, through newsletters and seminars, offers members information on consumer trends, networking resources, and perspectives into business solutions. More information on this organization can be found at CTFI's Web site (http://www.consumerexpert.org).

Focus Groups

Traditional focus groups are conducted with a group of neutral individuals who are not going to benefit directly from your service. When manufacturers are introducing a new product, they always conduct focus groups to get feedback. You can think the same way.

Suppose you have an idea: to offer a nutrition series for new parents. To determine whether this is a good idea, consider a pediatrician's staff your focus group. Ask if you can get their opinion on your idea. Since members of focus groups expect to receive something in return for the time they spend with you, offer to provide the first class to them as a thank you for serving as your focus group.

Perhaps you want to develop educational materials for the athletes you counsel. After you do a Web-based computer search to determine the resources already in print on this topic, take your idea directly to the athletes. Call your local roadrunners group. Offer to give a lecture; in return, have the participants evaluate your ideas.

Volunteer to give a free lecture to a group of senior citizens residing in a retirement community. In return, gather feedback on an idea to provide "cooking for one" classes. Those attending your seminar have just served as your focus group. The only cost to you is the time you spend doing a lecture.

Advisory Boards

Ask a health care provider, your mentor, and a client to serve as your advisory board. Have an informal brainstorming session at a convenient time and location. Offer to buy them breakfast in return for serving as your advisory board for your newly formed practice. Find out what they think is lacking in the community, get their input on your office location, find out what they think is reasonable for you to charge for your services. Your advisory board will be flattered to be a part of your business venture.

The Service or Product You Are Selling

Marketing a product that is tangible will be somewhat different from marketing a professional service that is intangible. The information that follows is about service marketing, although you will find that many strategies are similar.

Successful marketing requires a "hook," something that makes you or your practice unique (1). In *Guerilla Marketing: Secrets For Making Big Profits From Your Small Business,* Jay Levinson writes, "People do not pay attention to advertising. They pay attention only to things that interest them" (6). Think about what will attract people. When physicians decide to refer a patient to you, they are interested in only one thing: how you will help the patient. Although your resume may be impressive, the resume is not what helps the patient.

Your hook can be your unique approach, your success rate, or your office hours. To define your marketing hook, start by developing a mission statement about your practice. In your mission statement, include who you are, how you can help the patient, and a brief summary of your philosophy. Once complete, who you are will become clearer to your target population. How you are different from your competition will also be highlighted. Be honest and up front about your philosophy. Don't hide behind your philosophy, regardless of how unconventional it might be. Just be sure that your statement reflects you. That is what will separate you from the pack. For assistance in creating a mission statement, refer to Box 5.3.

Developing a niche and marketing to that niche can be beneficial. Your niche could be a specific clinical area, such as diabetes, food allergies, or vegetarians. Or it could be a certain age group, such as elderly persons or children. Or it might be developed based on special skills you possess, such as your fluency in Spanish, your geographic location, or your willingness to do home visits.

Marketing to a niche automatically targets your marketing efforts. For instance, if you are a certified diabetes educator, then focusing your market-

---

BOX 5.3

**WHO OR WHAT ARE YOU MARKETING:
FORMULATING A MISSION STATEMENT**

People form impressions of others within the first twenty to thirty seconds. It is critical that you prepare your personal "promotion" and mission statement. Plan what you will say. The preparation you do will help you to get better results in all your marketing activities.

Using 20 words or less, describe who you are and what you do:

_____

_____

_____

Using 20 words or less, describe how your services will benefit the consumer:

_____

_____

_____

ing campaign on endocrinologists, internists, and other dietitians will generate a specific clientele.

Your market may be overweight individuals; however, a focus on a particular segment of that population will help you with more specific marketing. The tools you might use to market to overweight middle-aged executives, for example, will be quite different from the tools you will use to market to overweight teenagers. For actual examples of niche marketing, refer to Box 5.4.

BOX 5.4
TRUE EXAMPLES OF NICHE MARKETING

- "I primarily see cancer patients, a natural specialization for me since I have spent the last 13 years working in oncology at the University of Colorado Hospital four days a week. My frustration with the lack of outpatient services available to cancer patients drove me to set up a private practice on my day off! I was asked to give a talk for the local oncology nursing group. The rep sponsoring it was very happy with the response, and I have since given other talks for her. After speaking to our local dietetics group last May, I was asked to join the speaker's bureau for Ross and Novartis, and did training for Ross. I've loved this aspect of working with cancer patients/providers and it pays well! It has proven to be a great way to market my private practice." (Colleen Gill, MS, RD)

- "I believe I have a niche in nutrient analysis and food labeling. My customers have included Costco Wholesale, *O* Magazine, LSG Sky Chefs, Rodale Press (cookbooks), a small Vermont food producer, and fellow RDs who write or cook but don't do the analysis piece for recipes." (Wendy Hess, RD, CDE)

- "I specialize in maternal health, mainly dealing with pregnant women, healthy or with gestational diabetes, and postpartum women. I do both nutrition counseling and fitness classes designed for prenatal and postpartum. I chose this niche as I felt it was important to become an expert in a particular population. I chose pregnant women because I thought, 'well, at least this group will listen to what I tell them.' Also, I had just had a baby and was totally in love with my baby and being pregnant, so I had an immediate interest in the subject." (Maria Pari-Keener, MS, RD)

Generalist or Specialist?

As you market your services, you will want to determine whether you are going to market yourself as a generalist or as a specialist (7). A generalist practice will allow you to see a wide range of clients. Generalists need to be current and informed about all that is trendy and be prepared for change. Generalists will rarely get stale or bored.

As a specialist, you will be providing services in an area about which you feel passionately, and where you have a great deal of knowledge. Your specialty may be what separates you from your competition. However, you have to work extremely hard to stay current in other areas.

Dietetics professionals question whether a general practice or a specialized practice is right for them. The answer is, "It depends." Over time your practice may evolve. Although you might know the answer from the start, it is likely that the answer will emerge as you begin to practice. For further guidance on this issue, see Box 5.5 (7).

BOX 5.5

GENERALIST OR SPECIALIST?

Specialized Practice

Specializing your practice makes good sense if you have a passion for a specific area of nutrition or if you would like to offer one particular type of service or MNT to your clients.

Pros
- If you specialize in one or two areas you are passionate about, you can focus on working with clients within your realm of interest.
- You have a greater depth of information in a given area than the vast majority of other dietitians.
- You have likely gathered abundant resources within your specialty, which will simplify staying abreast of changes in your area.
- If you live in a market with many other nutritionists, a specialty practice will set you apart.
- Specialists can usually charge more than generalists.
- Specialists draw from a larger geographic area, as people will travel a greater distance to see a specialist.
- If you are the only one in your community specializing in your area, it will minimize competition.

Cons

- There may not be a great enough need with your area of practice to create full-time employment.

- You can become outdated in other areas of nutrition very quickly. (E.g., if your food allergy client has diabetes and you have not kept up with the latest in diabetes management, you would need to refer him elsewhere.)

- You may incur greater continuing education costs if local CPE opportunities do not pertain to your area of interest and you must travel greater distances to meet your educational needs.

- Membership in specialty professional organizations may be more expensive (e.g., Food Allergy Network, American Academy of Allergy, Asthma and Immunology, etc.).

- If other local practitioners specialize in your area, competition will exist. Do a SWOT analysis (Strengths, Weaknesses, Opportunities and Threats) for you and your competitors.

Flexible Practice

If you don't have a specific area of interest or you enjoy the challenge of keeping current with a broader base of nutrition specialties, creating a more flexible practice may better suit your needs. However, are you confident that you have the energy and expertise to do everything, including MNT and more?

Pros

- You can consistently use and hone a broad range of skills including coaching, counseling, business, fitness, marketing, public speaking, teaching, and writing.

- You can keep your approach fresh by dabbling in many different areas.

- Your business can constantly change and evolve as new opportunities arise or needs surface.

- Having a wide area of expertise gives you access to a broader base of clients, which is important in starting a business.

- Frequent new challenges are intellectually stimulating.

Cons

- Keeping current with nutrition updates in many different specialty areas may be challenging.

- If you only have traditional experience, you may need additional training.

- Even if you have previous experience, you may still need to fine tune skills.

- There may be several RDs in flexible practice in your area which increases competition. Do a SWOT analysis (Strengths, Weaknesses, Opportunities, and Threats) for you and your competitors.

Source: Reprinted with permission from ADA Nutrition Entrepreneurs. *Nutrition Entrepreneurs Tool Kit: Specialized or Flexible Practice?* Chicago, Ill: ADA Nutrition Entrepreneurs; 2001. http://www.nedpg.org.

For many reasons, it might be necessary to see all types of patients when you first start your private practice. As your practice grows, you might find that you have a knack for working with an aging population, or you might get frustrated and annoyed when working with children. Try working with many populations. What you love will emerge, and it will most likely be what you are good at.

Pricing your services needs to be a part of your marketing plan. Determining the price you should charge for your services is covered in Chapter 4. From a marketing standpoint, it never makes sense to market yourself based on price. Marketing on price can devalue the quality of your service. You do not want potential clients to choose to see you simply because you are the least expensive. Although price may be a factor when someone is deciding whether to "purchase" your service, it is better business sense to market based on other factors, such as success rate, philosophy, or expertise.

Tools and Methods for Reaching Your Target Market

Potential clients will know of your services through your marketing efforts. The goal in marketing is simple: get your name out and keep it out in a cost-effective way. There are many tools available to you for marketing. When selecting marketing tools and strategies, you will need to consider your market. The tools you use may be different if you are marketing to a health club, a physicians' practice, or a consumer group in the community. Focus on what seems appropriate to the market and what will be the most cost-effective.

There are four general categories for promoting your services: networking, advertising, publicity, and word of mouth. Finding the right mix of promotional activities to get your name out and keep it out in an affordable way is your goal (1,3,5,8).

Networking: It's Not What You Know . . . It's Who You Know

Networking is defined as "the process of 'working' with or contacting others in order to achieve objectives or goals" (9). New entrepreneurs are sometimes uncomfortable with the concept of networking. Some view it as using people. True networking, however, is building personal relationships that are mutually beneficial. It is about giving *and* receiving.

Networking is not simply going to an event, handing out your business card, and collecting other people's business cards. Networking requires you to have a plan to connect with others, to share information, and to receive something in return to further your professional or personal goals (10,11).

FINDING YOUR NETWORKS

Any situation where you can meet people, share your vision, gather information from the group, and hopefully offer them something in return is a network. You can start by creating a list of your existing networks. This list should include your personal and professional acquaintances. Your personal networks could include your relatives, your children's school, your place of worship, your softball team, and your community association.

Your professional networks include your colleagues at work (if you are still employed), dietetic organizations, other health professionals such as doctors and therapists, organizations such as college alumni groups, and civic organizations.

In addition to the ADA, you will want to join and become an active member in other professional organizations where you can meet a targeted audience. Just being a member of an organization is not networking. Being an active member means you give and get. Dietetic practice groups, health organizations such as the American Diabetes Association, and professional organizations such as the National Speakers Bureaus will provide an opportunity to share and learn from others with similar interests and goals.

Remember to network with competitors. One of the best existing networks is other dietitians. Dietitians new to private practice fear that dietetics professionals with established practices will perceive them as competition. However, other dietitians can be an excellent referral source for you. Get to know about their practices so that when you get a referral you cannot handle, you can reciprocate. Referring to others is an important aspect of doing business.

STRATEGIES FOR NETWORKING

Learning how to network is an art. Attend professional meetings, social gatherings, and even family events with a networking frame of mind. Don't wait for people to seek you out. You must make the effort to get to know your networks. Think about who your networks are, and put yourself in a position to be active within those networks. If you are focusing your practice on diabetes management, become active in the local American Diabetes Chapter. If you are specializing in geriatrics, look at networking opportunities offered through AARP.

Take advantage of your membership in organizations and the networking opportunities available. Professional organizations, including the American Dietetic Association, offer formal networking events. Toastmasters and business and civic groups also provide formal networking classes.

Every time you attend a meeting, a social gathering, or even a family dinner, you can network. Set a networking goal for yourself for each event you attend. Networking goals can include meeting a new person, providing a referral or resource, and following up with a new contact within five days of the networking event.

Make your Rolodex meaningful by keeping names memorable. When you meet someone, use the back of their business card to jot down something about your meeting to make them memorable. It could be a shared birthdate, their recent promotion, or their love of baseball. Rely on this when you reconnect. People will be impressed that you've taken an interest in them. They are more likely to share.

Do not attend a function with a negative attitude. If you get caught in a conversation that is not productive, excuse yourself. Avoid toxic people. They will not be helpful to building your network.

Invite conversation by practicing a welcoming introduction. Think of ways to encourage people to tell you about them. This is relationship building. It may take many introductions and exposures before people remember who you are. Come up with ten items you can share with someone. Use key words to make it easier for people to remember you. Refer to Box 5.6 for guidance (12).

BOX 5.6
DEVELOP A POWERFUL SELF-INTRODUCTION

Answer the following questions to develop an effective self-introduction:

- What do I love most about what I do?
- What do I want people to know about me?
- What is the value of what I offer?

Key phrases for introductions:

- I love helping people . . .
- I make sure my clients . . .
- I am dedicated to . . .
- I love working with . . . to . . .

Source: Adapted from Fisher D. *People Power: Twelve Power Principles to Enrich Your Business, Career, and Personal Networks.* Austin, Texas: Bard & Stephen Press; 1995:114-117, with permission from the author. Copyright © Donna Fisher.

Networking is about exposure and having fun. Plan to network at least once a week in a variety of settings. Networking can include lunch with a colleague or a power walk with a friend. Always follow up a formal or informal networking function with a note, an e-mail, or a phone call thanking the person for their efforts in helping you increase your network. For more networking tips, refer to Box 5.7 (10).

BOX 5.7
PRACTICE MAKES PERFECT

- **Make names memorable.** When you meet new people, don't rush introductions. Repeat their names and associate them with something that will make them easy to recall. Repeat your name a few times, too.

- **Invite conversation.** When asked what you do, practice your marketing lines. Answer succinctly. Explain in a way that shows what you do and encourages conversation.

- **Business cards are not handbills.** The number of cards you hand out doesn't measure successful networking. Instead, pour your energy into each conversation and exchange cards when necessary.

- **Network with competitors.** Get to know and trust your competition so you can refer business that's not in your area of expertise. Everyone wins.

- **Have fun.** It is fine to network in informal settings! If you look like you enjoy what you do, people will be more inclined to refer to you. Sell your passion.

- **Say thanks.** Look for appropriate yet creative ways to express appreciation to people who've helped you. Always offer to pay the tab if you've networked over a meal. A fruit basket, a bouquet of flowers, a massage. At a minimum, always send a thank you note.

- **Finish with the future in mind.** End conversations with people imagining they will be in your circle for years. Make dates to explore how you can help each other.

Source: Reprinted from Waymon L, Baber A. No-nonsense marketing. *Your Company.* 1993(Summer):37, with permission from the authors. Copyright © 1993 Lynne Waymon and Anne Baber, the authors of *Make Your Contacts Count* (New York, NY: AMA; 2002). For more information: see the Web site http://www.contactscount.com or call 301/589-8633.

Anyone you meet is potentially resourceful to you. Learning how and when to massage those connections is important. Practice a subtle but direct approach. Asking someone "What can you do for me?" is a turnoff. Craft your questions carefully. For example, ask: "Who else should I speak with?" There will be times when it is not appropriate to network . . . and there will be situations where you might not be interested in networking!

Networking is an ongoing activity. For as long as you are in business, you will need to keep your networks alive. Always be "on." You never know who that person in line at the grocery store may be.

Advertising

Good advertising means getting the word out often. For advertising to be effective, the message must be repeated several times. There are plenty of low-cost advertising tools. Regardless of which you use, two basic advertising concepts must be employed: it must be catchy and it must be repeated (1,2,5). Refer to Box 5.8 for further advice on marketing.

BOX 5.8
MARKETING WORDS OF WISDOM BY LYNN KLETZKIN

---

1. If you can't describe your service in five seconds, you've already lost a potential client.

2. Change is constant; recognize new lifestyles and trends.

3. Your service is only as good as the consumer confidence you build around it.

4. Client perception is everything.

5. A better way always exists; be tenacious about your creativity.

6. What was good this year is not good enough for next year.

7. Get new ideas from your clients.

8. How you relate to and treat your clients is sometimes more important than your service.

9. Think BIG! It's just as much work as thinking small.

10. If you believe in your service but can't get a foot in the door, invest in a marketing counselor to get you started. Time is money.

When you are starting out, choose the most appropriate medium and upgrade as you can afford it. Advertising allows you to control your message. Take the time to plan a well-designed ad. If you can't afford to have it professionally designed, have it evaluated by friends and colleagues. Take their input seriously, and revise your advertising until the message is presented in a clear, concise, and catchy way.

NEWSPAPERS

Newspapers can be good advertising tools, although some can be very costly. If you live in a large metropolitan area, use a small, community-based newspaper. It will be more affordable and will reach a more targeted audience.

Think carefully about ad placement. If your paper has a health edition or food edition, placing an ad in that section will reach an already interested audience. If you are focusing on sports nutrition, have your ad placed on the sports page. Some newspapers offer "bulletin boards," which advertise classes, community events, or lectures. This is free advertising. If you can, be sure to take advantage of this opportunity.

When planning your newspaper ad, remember to budget for several releases. Good advertising needs to appear several times. A one-time newspaper ad will likely not generate the attention you want. Also, do not forget to design your ad so that it is punchy and informative.

YELLOW PAGES

Advertising in the yellow pages is targeted to a captive audience. The person searching the yellow pages has already determined they need to "buy" that service. It is generally inexpensive to place an ad. If you have a business telephone, you might be entitled to a free listing. Consider placing your ad in several different categories. For example, weight loss, nutrition specialist, and sports may all be appropriate ad placement categories.

The yellow pages do not have stated criteria for who can advertise, so you might find yourself competing with large diet centers or unlicensed professionals. Think carefully about what type of client you want to attract and advertise with that in mind.

NONPRINT MEDIA: TELEVISION AND RADIO

Airtime, regardless of the market, is expensive. A paid commercial is probably out of the budget for most dietetics professionals just starting out. If you are trying to advertise an event as opposed to your own practice, networks and radio stations may offer the opportunity for a public service announcement. Exposure and name recognition are important, so do not pass up this opportunity if it exists.

THE INTERNET

Many dietetics professionals think they must have a Web site to be "cutting edge." Having a Web site to be able to communicate better with your potential or existing clients, to sell a product or service, or to establish credibility in the marketplace are some reasons why dietitians create Web sites. Developing, maintaining, and promoting a Web site can be costly. Should you choose to have a Web site, you will need to decide whether you will build it yourself or hire a professional. You will also need to decide who will host the Web site. Think through your purpose and your target audience before committing time and resources to developing one (13).

If you cannot afford a Web site, you can still use the Internet as a marketing tool. When using e-mail, always have a signature that provides complete contact information (14). This is free advertising every time you send an e-mail. Take advantage of this.

DIRECT MAIL

Direct mail includes any promotional piece that connects directly with the consumer. There are many options available to you, each with its unique selling power. Direct mail includes post cards, brochures, flyers, announcements, and newsletters. Even a follow-up letter to a referring physician is a form of direct mail.

Targeted mailing lists can be purchased from several different organizations. If you are mailing to other dietetics professionals to promote a class or product, mailing lists can be purchased from the ADA and targeted for geographic region or by specialty area. Other professional organizations sell lists, too. Your local medical society may be a good source if you are mailing to physicians or other health professionals.

Once your target group is identified, think about what other services they may use to access an existing mailing list. If it is for a class for new parents, think about the products all new parents will be purchasing, and contact that source to see if a list is available. You can also generate your own mailing list for free by accessing your e-mail address book and your Rolodex.

BROCHURES

A printed brochure allows you to go into detail about your services. Brochures can be excellent marketing tools and relatively inexpensive to create. To keep costs down, brochures can be created on a computer. Important elements to highlight would be your location, your philosophy, and what makes your service unique. It's also nice to "give something away" on the brochure, such as a sample recipe or a healthy eating tip.

When designing the brochure, always keep the audience in mind. For example, a brochure designed to send to other professionals may have a different look from a brochure you will be distributing at a health club. Your brochure should look professional and should help you to establish credibility. For further guidance, refer to Box 5.9.

BOX 5.9
GUIDELINES FOR DEVELOPING A BROCHURE

1. Identify your audience. This determines the tone of your brochure. For the dietetics professional in private practice, two broad audiences are

   - the general public.

   - referring health professionals.

2. Consider the purpose of the brochure. It could be

   - to distribute at lectures.

   - to mail to prospective clients.

   - to mail to referral sources, such as physicians, therapists, or schools.

3. Keep samples of brochures that you like. It is easier to identify features you like and don't like and to adapt them to accommodate your unique practice than to create a brochure from scratch. If a professional will be assisting you, bring the brochures with you.

4. Make a "dummy" brochure by folding paper and laying out items.

5. Brochures are generally 8.5 X 11.5 or 8.5 X 14 inches. They need to be folded to fit into a business envelope for mailing.

6. Brochures are generally divided into three panels, using the front and the back of the paper.

   - One panel is used for the headlines. This is where you prominently display information about yourself: name, credentials, address, telephone number, e-mail address, Web site URL. You would also put your logo here, if you have one. This is what your audience will read first. It should move the reader to call you.

(continues)

BOX 5.9 (CONTINUED)

- One panel is where you describe your services. Emphasize how you will help a prospective patient, how someone will benefit from your services, and how your services are unique. Perhaps you perform computerized dietary analysis or measure metabolic rates. These are unique features to highlight. Establish your credibility by stating your success rate, if possible.

- One panel is where you might give away advice, such as a recipe, include testimonials (get permission), and insert your picture (optional).

7. Make sure the language you use is simple. This is not the place to be clinical or show off your vocabulary. Use the active voice when writing and avoid clichés. Choose simple words, which will excite people and motivate them to call you.

8. The typeface you select must be reader friendly. There are three main families of typeface: cursive, serifs, and sans serif. In general, serif is easiest to read. Do not mix typefaces, because it usually detracts from the overall look of the brochure and makes it more difficult to read.

9. The quality of the paper you use is determined by your budget. Use the best you can afford, but your money will be better spent on the creative portion and developing snappy copy.

10. Let your personal style show through, even if a professional is designing it for you.

ANNOUNCEMENTS

Announcements are most successful when you are established and have something new to announce. For example, a new partner, a new location, or a new program might be appropriate reasons to send an announcement. There are likely better ways to spend your marketing budget than sending announcements out to let people know you have opened a new practice. Since your name won't be recognized, the person you wish to reach may never read the announcement before it is tossed in the trash. For a generic announcement, see Figure 5.1.

FIGURE 5.1

Generic announcement.

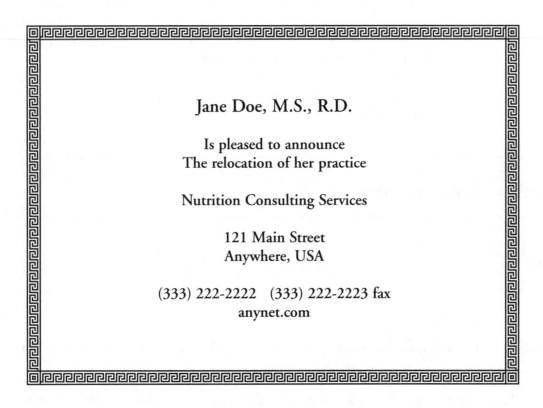

Jane Doe, M.S., R.D.

Is pleased to announce
The relocation of her practice

Nutrition Consulting Services

121 Main Street
Anywhere, USA

(333) 222-2222   (333) 222-2223 fax
anynet.com

FLYERS

Flyers can be an inexpensive and creative way to advertise. They are similar to brochures in that they allow you to discuss your service in a more personal way. A well-designed flyer can promote a professional image. Distribute them with thought. Rather than leaving your flyers on car windshields, strategically place them on community bulletin boards, a physician's office waiting area, or as a give-away at a local road race. Just be sure to ask permission before distributing them. To make them meaningful, include fast-food facts, holiday tips, or even a recipe of the month. Be sure the flyer includes the important information about you and your practice.

FOLLOW-UP LETTERS AND THANK-YOU NOTES

An overlooked piece of direct mail is the follow-up letter you send to a physician or a thank-you note you send to a referral source. (*Important note:* You must have your patients sign a release to allow you to do this. Refer to Chapter 3 for more information on client privacy issues.) Follow-up letters are direct mail pieces with very targeted and receptive audiences. You might also include an article that appeared in the newspaper or in a newsletter on a relevant nutrition topic. The name of the game in advertising is to keep your name out there. Always include business cards and a flyer or a brochure, if possible. For a sample follow-up letter, see Box 5.10.

BOX 5.10

SAMPLE FOLLOW-UP LETTER

Date

Re:_____

Dear_____,

Thank you for allowing me the pleasure of seeing this patient for medical nutrition therapy. _____came to see me concerning _____.

_____stands _____ tall and weighs _____ pounds, with a body mass index (BMI) of _____. His/her healthy weight range is _____ to _____, with a BMI of _____.

A complete nutrition assessment indicated to me that _____
_____.

I reviewed this with _____ and provided him/her with a written summary of these findings. Together we established goals for medical nutrition therapy.

A follow-up appointment has been scheduled in _____weeks time.

Thank you again for this kind referral.

Sincerely,

_____, R.D.

Additional comments:

HOLIDAY CARDS AND GIFTS

Sending holiday cards to your referral sources and to your client base is direct mail advertising. It is another way of keeping your name out there. Purchase or design cards that reflect you and your practice. Add a personal note at the bottom. Also consider sending holiday gifts to referral sources. A fruit basket, a nice cookbook, or a subscription to a health newsletter are all appreciated gifts.

Debra Rutenberg, a promotional marketing associate at The AdSolution in Rockville, MD, suggests sending cards and gifts after the first of the year. They will stand out and be remembered (oral communication, November 2003). Do not forget National Nutrition Month as an opportunity for marketing your services, by sending a gift, an article, or a card.

NEWSLETTERS

Although a newsletter is a great way to advertise, it should not be the first tool to be used for advertising your business. Creating and publishing a newsletter is time consuming and expensive. It can be added to your "bag of tricks" when you are looking to grow and diversify your business. For an example of a newsletter, see Figure 5.2 on page 126.

PROFESSIONAL DIRECTORIES

There are two ways to advertise in directories. One is as a member of an organization, and the other is by actually placing an ad for your service in the directory. Being a member of different professional organizations often comes with the benefit of having your name published in their directory. Your dietetic practice group or the local chapter of the American Heart Association or of Women in Business may have directories that will reach different populations.

Medical societies often publish directories for physicians and other health professionals. If your medical community publishes a directory but does not include dietitians in it, suggest that they add the section. It will make their directory more complete.

Remember to think of all your networks: your child's school, your garden club, your place of worship. Do they publish a directory? Is it your target audience? If so, advertise in it. Directories can be a very inexpensive form of advertising. Sometimes a reprint of your business card can take the place of a formal ad.

FIGURE 5.2

Example of a newsletter. *Tiny Tummies.* 2003;8(10):1. Reprinted with permission from Tiny Tummies. Copyright © 2003.

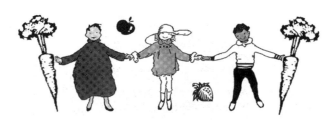

Tiny Tummies™

Good Food for Growing Families

Volume IX, Issue 6   November/December 2003

Eat Well, Spend Less

Eating well and trying to save on groceries means balancing time with money and flavor with convenience. It is a challenge for every family. Consider also the costs and benefits of food choices as they affect your family lifestyle, the people and economics in your community, and the environment. Saving money is one important goal and eating well is equally important. Here are some ideas to help you do both.

Find out how much you spend on food. Keep a record of your food costs for a month. Save receipts from every loaf of bread, every latte, every meal out. This will be your best tool for identifying where to cut.

Cook at home. Homemade food tastes better and usually costs less. The more you know about food and cooking, the easier and more enjoyable it is to get dinner on the table or to pack lunches. Buy the classic, comprehensive American cookbook, The Joy of Cooking. Read this newsletter. Attend a cooking class; whether it is Boiling Wa-

ter 101 or Advanced Thai Cuisine, you will learn valuable techniques to use every day. Watch TV cooking shows, keeping in mind that most are hosted by restaurant chefs, not home cooks. Ask your family and friends to share ideas and recipes.

Eat local food. It is usually less expensive than out-of-season fruit and vegetables shipped from points south. But saving tons of dough isn't the only goal. Eating food grown in your area is good for the local economy, saves the cost and environmental damage of long-distance shipping and keeps you connected to your community. Food has more flavor and meaning when it comes from local dirt. Farmer's markets and Community Sup-

ported Agriculture (CSA) are great, so is asking your grocer to stock local food.

Grow your own. You can't get more local than that. Teaching kids how vegetables and fruits are grown is priceless. For the same cost as a bunch of fresh herbs, buy a whole plant for a window box. A few pots on a balcony can save you lots on lettuce. For the price of a pound of green beans, grow as many as your family can eat. If you think food from the Farmer's Market tastes good, you will be astounded by your own.

Breastfeed. I guess this is the same as "growing your own!" Extra food for a nursing mother

(Continued on page 2)

In This Issue	*page*
Red Beans & Rice	3
Tiny Tummies' Guide to Breakfast Cereals	4
Teething Biscuits for Babies	5
Olives & Olive Oil	6
In Season: Winter Squash	8
A Little Thanksgiving History	9
Tiny Tummies' Food & Nutrition News	10

Tiny Tummies P.O. Box 5756, Napa CA, 94581 phone/fax: (707) 251-0550 TinyTummies.com Text Copyright 2003

1

Publicity

Publicity is basically free advertising. It includes anything that gets your name to the target population. It can be a quote you've given to a newspaper, an article you've written, or publicity flyers distributed for a talk you are giving. The downside to publicity is that, when you are interviewed, you lose the ability to control what is said about you. The interviewer can use your comments in any way they might fit into a story. Although reporters are not out to make you look bad, they do control what they write from the interview.

Your target market will view publicity as more credible than paid advertising. Readers often think that if an article features you or relies on you as an expert, or if you've been asked to speak to a group, then you must be credible. Publicity tends to have greater longevity than paid advertising. Readers will likely remember it better than advertising. The key is learning how to become noteworthy enough to attract good publicity.

PRESS RELEASES AND PRESS KITS

The first step in attracting publicity is to develop a press release. You can send a press release to anyone who might have any interest in what you are doing. Perhaps you have a new software program to analyze recipes, a new piece of equipment to measure percentage of body fat, or you are starting a cooking program for senior citizens. These could all seem newsworthy to the right media source.

When preparing a press release, make it punchy and short. One page, double-spaced is the maximum. Be sure to include relevant contact information. Make the press release memorable by being creative. The ordinary and mundane will not attract attention. For guidance on creating a press release, refer to Box 5.11.

BOX 5.11
GUIDELINES FOR CREATING A PRESS RELEASE

1. The content must be newsworthy. Your release must have an angle or "hook" to get read at all.

2. Start strong. Your first sentence and your first paragraph must tell the story. It should tell the reader the who, what, when, where, and why of the story. The reader may not read beyond that first sentence. Subsequent paragraphs can provide details.

(continues)

BOX 5.11 (continued)

3. Use the active voice. Avoid cliches and stick to the facts. Omit unnecessary adjectives and make each word meaningful. Every word counts.

4. Include a release date at the top of the press release. FOR IMMEDIATE RELEASE should appear at the top of your press release.

5. Do not use exclamation points. They add nothing to a press release.

6. Never use all upper-case letters or type in bold (except for the IMMEDIATE RELEASE at the top of the page).

7. Press releases are not used to make sales. They should not scream "buy me."

8. Be sure to include your complete contact information.

9. Proofread and check grammar.

A press kit should be created if you plan on promoting yourself to the media or to organizations interested in hiring you for speaking. Your press kit should include a bio or resume, a copy of media work, published writing samples if available, a brochure if you have one, any information on your services including testimonials, and a photograph of yourself.

You can develop a simple press kit without professional help. There are numerous programs and Web sites that will help you get started. However, if your goal is to attract a national presence, you will need to invest the money to have a professional press kit created.

WRITE AN ARTICLE

Having a byline and getting published is great publicity. Although many dietitians will get paid for writing, others will write for the name recognition or as a stepping-stone to larger projects. If you are writing for free, negotiate for free advertising space in return for writing an article.

Writing takes time, talent, and drive. You do not need to start with a large daily newspaper to be published. Think about what your target market reads. Perhaps you are working with the pediatric population. Writing for a locally produced parenting magazine or newspaper, or even contributing an article for the local Parent-Teacher Association (PTA) would provide you with exposure to your target population. If your interest is in sports nutrition, find a local fitness center with a monthly newsletter, and volunteer to write an article. Or perhaps you are interested in conducting supermarket tours. If so, see if your local supermarket chain might be interested in having you write a column for their newsletter.

If you do not have the time or interest to write an article, find a relevant article written by someone else. Let the reader know that you are a local expert on that topic. Be sure to request permission to have it reprinted. (Costs for reprint permissions vary extensively. Some might be free of charge; others can be quite expensive.)

GET QUOTED: BECOME THE EXPERT

To become the local expert, you will need to develop relationships with the local media. Learning how to work with the media is an art that is not mastered overnight. Offer yourself as an expert by sending them a press release about a program you are doing in the community, by providing them with a press kit including information about your practice, or just by calling them to respond to a story they did. The media will appreciate your availability as a credible source rather than as a dietetics professional who is trying to get her name in print (15).

Reporters appreciate hearing about story ideas. However, not all ideas are considered. For serious consideration, a story idea should be unique, topical, or present a new angle on a previously covered topic. If one reporter is not interested in the topic, ask if he or she is aware of someone who might be interested. Be persistent, but do not be a pest (16).

Generally, reporters always need the information yesterday. If a reporter calls you, be sure to respond in a timely way. Often, the reporter will use the first person that returns their call. If you know the time and topic of the interview, be prepared. If you are not prepared with an answer when a reporter calls, ask if you can return the call in 15 minutes. In that time, collect your thoughts. Have a few important "sound bites" of information. Limit your answers to the questions asked. The more you talk to reporters, the more comfortable you will become asking them to repeat what you've said, to minimize the risks of being misquoted. Follow up promptly with supporting information requested. If you don't know the topic, the best thing you can do is to provide them with the name of someone who does.

Realize that this process can be frustrating. You might provide 45 minutes of your time and in return receive a two-second sound bite or a one-sentence quote. Sometimes you might receive no mention at all. Follow up by contacting the writer after the article has appeared. Give them feedback. Thank the reporter for including your information or for consulting with you, even if you were not mentioned.

Notice when dietetics professionals are quoted, contact them, and ask them how they became a resource to the media. If a dietitian has a relationship with the media, advise her of your expertise. Professionals should recognize their limitations and, if they are aware of your expertise, may refer the media to you. Refer to Box 5.12 for additional help on this subject (16).

BOX 5.12
WORKING WITH THE MEDIA

- If news breaks in your area of expertise, let reporters know you're available to answer their questions.

- Once you establish rapport with reporters and they realize you are a source of accurate information, they will call you back for future stories.

- Package your message creatively and then pitch it to a reporter as a story idea.

- A radio audience must "visualize" your message mentally, so it's especially important to speak clearly and use words that conjure pictures.

- Visual impact sells a television story, so add a visual dimension to your message. For an interview on portion distortion, you might bring "super sized" products and compare them to more "normal" portions.

- Always ask about and respect a reporter's deadline. If you know you can't respond in time for a reporter's deadline, say so at the start.

- Send reporters follow-up notes after an interview to acknowledge a well-written article or an effective broadcast story.

Source: Adapted from Nowlin B. Keep it short and simple: how to master the "sound bite" and other tips for crafting effective media messages about nutrition. *J Am Diet Assoc:* 1994;94:971-973, with permission from Elsevier. Copyright © 1994 American Dietetic Association.

GIVE TALKS OR PRESENTATIONS

Name recognition and keeping your name visible are the cornerstones of marketing. One easy way to do this is to make yourself available for speaking engagements. Nutrition is a topic of interest to almost everyone. Learning how to speak publicly to different audiences is important. Research your audience before giving the talk. Do not focus on selling your services to the audience. If you do a good job, the audience members may request a card. Also, be sure to have handouts available when you speak. And, of course, always include contact information.

One way to get started locally is to call groups of physicians in your target market. Offer to provide lunchtime in-service on a relevant topic. The latest dieting trends, restaurant eating guidelines, or holiday eating tips will appeal to those in the office and to the patients they serve. Your goal is for the referring sources to see you as the expert. However, even if the referring physicians don't show up for the in-service, getting your name known by office personnel is often just as helpful. For examples of presentation topics, see Box 5.13.

BOX 5.13

HOT TOPICS FOR IN-SERVICES

January:	How to keep those New Year's resolutions
February:	The latest thoughts on Heart Health
March:	National Nutrition Month . . . know your dietetics professionals
April:	Getting ready for summer . . . comparison of latest diet trends
May:	Fast food choices
June:	Supplement safety
July:	Picnic safety
August:	Back to school lunch
September:	Satisfying snack foods
October:	Yikes . . . it's Halloween
November:	Eating well when eating out
December:	Navigating your way through the holiday season

Ask the office if you can provide the in-service at lunch, and offer to bring food. The money spent on catering lunch for a small, busy office will be much more targeted than mailing an announcement, which may never get read by the right person.

Join speakers' bureaus, such as the National Speakers Bureau (http://www.speaker.org), or the speakers' bureaus of your professional organizations. You will learn how to be a better speaker and, with some marketing, can be called upon as a speaker.

VOLUNTEER AT HEALTH FAIRS

Many organizations conduct health fairs. If the health fair is reaching your target audience, it is a good way to get your name out and earn credibility. Although a health fair unrelated to your target population is unlikely to bring you business, it is a good way to practice speaking with an audience that you probably will not address again. Suggestions for health fairs might include trying out a new topic, inviting participants to test your new nutrient analysis program, or creating a new tip sheet and getting feedback.

COMMUNITY INVOLVEMENT

Investigate the possibilities of donating a free consultation to a targeted auction or community event. Schools, places of worship, and charitable organizations may hold an auction to raise funds. Auction catalogues and publicity for the event will serve as your free advertising. You can give back to your community and receive free publicity for your service.

WORD OF MOUTH

A satisfied customer is your best marketing tool. You can't control this free advertising, but it works the best. Being competent, caring for your client base, and a little luck with satisfied clients is what will ultimately promote your services.

Marketing: A Summary

"It takes money to make money." You need to determine not whether you can afford marketing but how much you can spend on marketing to get the biggest bang for your buck. Be realistic. Very few dietetics professionals will be able to foot the bill for a large marketing campaign. That does not mean you should forgo marketing. It simply means you need to do your research and invest your money where you will reap the biggest returns. Marketing dollars must be spent wisely. The effectiveness of marketing needs to be constantly monitored. As discussed above, there are less expensive ways to market—seek out these opportunities. Advertising allows you to control the message but is more costly. Publicity and word of mouth, although free, do not allow you to control the message, only to influence it.

Marketing is a dynamic process. You do not create a marketing plan, try it out, and go into business. From the inception of your business until you retire, you need to be marketing, reevaluating, and revising the marketing as needed. Marketing should be fun and should allow you and your business to shine.

Evaluate your marketing knowledge and get professional help where you feel inadequate. Tap into free services offered through organizations including the ADA and the Small Business Administration, your local chamber of commerce, and public libraries.

Draw up a plan, think creatively, and go for it.

Keep the following vital points in mind:

- The 4 *P*s of marketing are product, place, price, and promotion. These all come together in the essential marketing plan.
- Analyzing your target market will help you to learn about the people who will buy your services. It should also reveal information about your competition. Knowing your competition is important in defining your own practice and in marketing your services.
- Successful marketing requires a "hook." Think about all the things that are unique about you and the services you offer. Location, hours, payment, philosophy, and niche are examples that can be used in a marketing campaign to make you look unique.
- Networking is essential to your success. Find out where your networks exist and learn how and when to network effectively.
- Advertising needs to be repeated to be meaningful. One-shot ads are generally not worth the investment.
- There are many different media, including newspapers, yellow pages, radio and television, the Internet, direct mail, brochures, announcements, flyers, follow-up letters, holiday cards, newsletters, and directories, which are available to you for advertising. Evaluate the cost, the image, and the effectiveness for your particular practice.
- Publicity is free advertising. You have little control over what is said about you, but it tends to give credibility to your services. To position yourself for publicity, create a press release or press kit, write an article, or offer your expertise to the media. Free publicity also comes

from giving talks, volunteering at health fairs, and being involved in your community.
- A satisfied client is the best form of advertising.

References

1. Tyson E, Schell J. *Small Business for Dummies.* New York, NY: John Wiley and Sons Publishing; 2003.
2. Levinson J, Godin S. *The Guerrilla Marketing Handbook.* New York, NY: Houghton Mifflin Company; 1994.
3. Marketing basics [United States Small Business Association Web site]. Available at: http://www.sba.gov/starting_business/marketing/basics.html. Accessed March 15, 2004.
4. American Dietetic Association Nutrition Entrepreneurs. *Nutrition Entrepreneurs Tool Kit: Marketing Your Services and Products.* Chicago, Ill: ADA Nutrition Entrepreneurs; 2001.
5. Pinson J, Jinnett J. *Steps to Small Business Start-Up. Everything You Need to Know to Turn Your Idea into a Successful Business.* Chicago, Ill: Dearborn Publishing; 2000.
6. Levinson J. *Guerrilla Marketing: Secrets for Making Big Profits from Your Small Business.* New York, NY: Houghton Mifflin Company; 1998.
7. American Dietetic Association Nutrition Entrepreneurs. *Nutrition Entrepreneurs Tool Kit: Specialized or Flexible Practice?* Chicago, Ill: ADA Nutrition Entrepreneurs; 2001.
8. Mintzer R. *The Everything Start Your Own Business Book.* Avon, Mass: Adams Media Corporation; 2002.
9. Byham-Gray L. Networking for success. *Today's Dietitian.* 2001;3:12–14.
10. Baber A, Waymon L. No-nonsense networking: a guide to cultivating new business contacts. *Your Company.* Summer 1993:34–38.
11. Lepke J. (Re)building a better career. *J Am Diet Assoc.* 1995;95:15–16.
12. Fisher D. *People Power: Twelve Power Principles to Enrich Your Business, Career, and Personal Networks.* Austin, Texas: Bard & Stephen Press; 1995.
13. Pangan T. Laying down the foundation of a successful Web site. *Ventures: Enterprising News and Ideas for Nutrition Entrepreneurs.* 2003;18:3–4.
14. Dorner B. Mega marketing skills for success. [Becky Dorner and Associates Web site]. Available at: http://www.beckydorner.com/pdf/MegaMarketingSkills.pdf. Accessed March 2, 2004.
15. McManamon B, Pazder N. Pitching your ideas to the media. *J Am Diet Assoc.* 2000;100:1451–1453.
16. Nowlin B. Keep it short and simple: how to master the "sound bite" and other tips for crafting effective media messages about nutrition. *J Am Diet Assoc:* 1994;94:971–973.

Chapter 6

Staying in Business

Attracting patients is your first goal in starting a private practice. Maintaining patients and growing your business is often secondary. There are standard business practices that should be used to achieve a thriving practice. A transition from the traditional role of nutrition educator to nutrition therapist needs to occur, to generate follow-up sessions, which, in business terms, translates into repeat business. This chapter will explore the necessary transitional changes that will enable you to create a successful nutrition practice.

From Educator to Counselor

It is projected that "in 2017, much [will have] changed since 2002: the role of the clinical dietitian [will] become that of a nutrition therapist." (1). Dietetics professionals employed in traditional settings, such as hospitals or outpatient clinics, have a difficult time envisioning the process in a private practice setting. Many dietetics professionals wonder: How do you structure your session? What do you do in follow-up sessions? How do you encourage patients to return? Answers to these questions cannot be readily apparent to the dietetics professional employed in a traditional setting.

Dietetics professionals are taught the medical model of patient care. This model is appropriate in hospital and clinical settings where dietetics professionals have historically practiced.

The traditional medical model relies on short-term nutrition intervention. The dietitian generates goals for the patient, focusing on what the patient needs to learn. Typically, the dietetics professional needs to develop only a superficial relationship with the patient. Nutrition counseling, using this model, includes assessing the patient's status, planning necessary diet changes, and then providing information. Counseling, in this sense, is really educating (2–4). Refer to Table 6.1 on page 136 for further detail about the nutrition therapy model (2).

TABLE 6.1

MEDICAL MODEL VS NUTRITION THERAPY MODEL

Medical Model	Nutrition Therapy Model
Short-term intervention primarily of an educational nature	Long-term care
Minimal relationship	A significant relationship in and of itself is a key part of the therapeutic process
Quickly determined, often standardized plan of action	A treatment plan that is highly individualized and evolves over time

Source: Data are from Reiff D, Reiff K. *Eating Disorders: Nutrition Therapy in the Recovery Process.* Gaithersburg, Md: Aspen Publishers; 1992.

Generally, when consulting inpatients, visits are brief. A diet consult may be requested when the patient is about to be discharged from a hospital. The patient may be preoccupied with other issues at this time. The consult may take place in a setting that is not private, so it is unlikely that the patient can be completely candid.

In an outpatient setting, you might have more time with the patient, but you still seize the opportunity to teach the patient instead of actual counseling, since you may never see the patient again. For the dietetics professional practicing in a clinical setting or in an outpatient department, the nutrition therapist rarely emerges. Rather, the dietetics professional serves a useful but quite different function as a nutrition educator.

Traditional dietetics counseling, by necessity, is very different from the process that can be used in a private practice setting. The process of nutrition therapy, more often used in a private practice, is a dynamic relationship between the dietetics professional and the patient and often between the dietetics professional and other health care providers. Refer to Table 6.2 for more information (2).

Nutrition therapy is a client-centered approach that focuses on beliefs, emotions, and behaviors. It results in forming a long-term relationship with your patients and with a psychotherapist if one is involved. Treatment plans are highly individualized and evolve over time (5).

Nutrition therapy, as a concept, is widely accepted in the eating disorders arena, and this approach is appropriate and necessary in most other

TABLE 6.2

COMPARING COUNSELING STYLES

Nutrition Education	Nutrition Therapy
Time constraints	More time
Gives dos and don'ts	Fosters choice among options
Limited rapport between dietitian and client	Dietitian and client develop a relationship
Limited follow-up	Open-ended
Client is dependent	Promotes client's independence
Less interdisciplinary coordination	Team approach is emphasized

Source: Adapted from Licavoli L. Dietetics goes into therapy. *J Am Diet Assoc.* 1995;95:751–752, with permission from Elsevier. Copyright © 1995 American Dietetic Association.

areas of patient counseling (4). Dietetics professionals learn that simply educating a client about dietary changes does not mean that the client will be able to implement the changes. To see real change with your patients, you will need to transition from being a nutrition educator to being a nutrition therapist.

Although some of your patients' goals will be accomplished merely by providing them with factual information, it is unlikely that you will be able to build a practice based on that. As your patients fail to make life-long changes, you will get frustrated and look for ways to help your patients become more successful. Making the transition will enable you to better help your patients. Your success will be measured by your clients' success. You will have more follow-up visits, and your satisfied clients will help you to build your practice.

Becoming a Nutrition Therapist

The transition from nutrition educator to nutrition therapist is a process that happens over time and through experience. The first part of the process is to understand basic counseling skills. The next phase is gradually using those skills in your practice. Most dietetics professionals are familiar with the counseling skills needed, but few may have the opportunity or confidence to use them.

Good Listening Skills

Our role as educators often preempts us from listening to our patients. We sometimes feel we don't have the time to listen. Listening to what clients actually want from the session is sometimes very different from what they need. Being a good listener will require you to be flexible in your approach. What you think a patient may be ready to address in your session may very well not be what they are ready to work on (6).

You may feel uncomfortable if there is silence in the room. There will be times when your response should be silence. You may be surprised by what you learn from your patient when you allow silence to fill the room. As awkward as it may seem initially, silence will help provide your patient with time to divulge more information. This process may be very valuable to the patient's overall success.

A good listener should be able to paraphrase what a patient says. This will allow the patient to have an opportunity to review the topics discussed in the session and can help clarify any misunderstandings.

Empathy and Support

When your patients respond to questions, you need to assume a nonjudgmental stance. They may never have felt safe enough to realize how food is so intertwined with the rest of their life and to talk openly about it. When patients realize that you are not there merely to provide the latest diet information, they may be more willing to share their feelings about the difficulty they face in making important and necessary diet changes. You can validate those feelings and be knowledgeable about how and when they can make any changes.

Care and Trust

Nutrition therapists must be caring and genuinely interested in helping their patients. These are attributes you cannot fake. Your patients must feel safe to talk freely about food and the issues around food. Listen to their concerns and respond in a caring manner. For a listing of what a patient looks for in a nutrition therapist, refer to Box 6.1 (2).

Dietetics professionals will benefit from formal counseling courses and from reading counseling books, but nothing will replace trying on different counseling styles with your patients. Counseling techniques can be labeled and defined, but becoming a nutrition therapist will be a result of actually using these techniques in practice. For a listing of helpful information, refer to Box 6.2.

BOX 6.1

WHAT PATIENTS WANT IN A NUTRITION THERAPIST

People with eating disorders want a nutrition therapist with the following traits:

- Is flexible

- Understands their fears about food and weight

- Will work at a pace they can handle

- Is caring and nonjudgmental

- Is patient

- Does not have unrealistic expectations

Source: Data are from Reiff D, Reiff K. *Eating Disorders: Nutrition Therapy in the Recovery Process.* Gaithersburg, Md: Aspen Publishers; 1992

BOX 6.2

RESOURCES FOR THE EMERGING NUTRITION THERAPIST

- *Moving Away from Diets,* by Karin Kratina, Nancy King, and Dayle Hayes. Published by Helm Seminars Publishing.

- Renfrew Center for Eating Disorders: Publishes quarterly newsletter addressing counseling topics. Holds annual symposium (http://www.renfrewcenter.com).

- MollyKellogg.com: Resource for supervision information and a monthly newsletter (http://www.mollykellogg.com).

- Sports Cardiovascular and Wellness Nutritionists (SCAN): Dietetic practice group with special interest in nutrition therapists (http://www.SCANdpg.org).

- Bulimia.com: A comprehensive listing of books, periodicals, and resources about treatment and prevention of eating disorders and other food issues (http://www.bulimia.com).

Two of ADA's dietetic practice groups, Sports, Cardiovascular, and Wellness Nutritionists (SCAN) and Nutrition Entrepreneurs (NE), have subunits to help practitioners develop their counseling skills. Dietitians working in the area of eating disorders have long appreciated the need to move beyond the traditional medical model. The following suggestions have been adapted from a tip sheet titled *Disordered Eating*, published by SCAN (7). While the tips offered are for expanding your work as a specialist in disordered eating, they are also useful to your development as a skilled counselor working with any population.

EXPAND YOUR STUDIES

Take a psychology class that includes information about personality disorders, cognitive behavioral interventions, family systems theory, and different counseling styles.

NETWORK

Discuss your interests with professors, colleagues, friends, and others who can enhance your knowledge in the field of eating disorders.

DO YOUR OWN PERSONAL WORK

You might want to discuss your own relationship to food, weight, exercise, and body image with a therapist. This work will give you the opportunity to experience what a counselor/client relationship is like and discover what techniques, approaches, and counseling styles you prefer.

CONSIDER SUPERVISION AND STAY CURRENT

Consider being supervised by a health professional you respect, one who has experience in working with eating-disordered patients. You can receive supervision from an experienced dietetics professional who specializes in eating disorders, a psychotherapist, or a physician.

Supervision is a concept widely used in the psychotherapy world. As dietitians, we may be unfamiliar with it. On her Web site, Molly Kellogg, RD, defines supervision as follows (8):

> When one or a group of nutrition therapists contract with an experienced professional to help them advance their counseling skills. It includes such things as: discussion of cases, exploration of the therapists' own issues that come up in client sessions, practice of new skills, advice on what to try next

with a particular client, support for limit-setting, handling burn-out, etc. The emphasis is on the *process* of counseling rather than on the content. It is assumed that participants have other sources of information on disease states, diet recommendations, etc.

As stated in the American Dietetic Association Code of Ethics, "The dietetics practitioner assumes responsibility and accountability for personal competence in practice, continually striving to increase professional knowledge and skills and to apply them in practice" (9). To advance as a nutrition therapist, supervision may be necessary and beneficial. As you collaborate more with mental health professionals, you will be able to identify those therapists whose work you admire, respect, and trust. It is appropriate to approach such therapists and inquire about supervision.

Dietetics professionals who are skilled nutrition therapists are available to provide supervision. Supervision is not mentoring. Although mentors do not expect reimbursement, when you engage in a professional supervision relationship with any health professional, you should expect to pay for that service.

Respect for Boundaries

As you move beyond the role of nutrition educator, you must be completely informed of ADA's Code of Ethics and Standards of Professional Practice (9,10). Behaviors play a role in how, what, why, and when we eat. Our work, as dietetics professionals, will always be grounded in food. To truly motivate a patient to change, the boundaries of nutrition therapy and psychotherapy will sometimes feel blurred. You should never assume that you are the psychotherapist . . . just the food therapist. You will need to have an understanding of what your domain is and what should be referred to a psychotherapist. If you are in a state that requires licensing, become familiar with the scope of practice. Always be knowledgeable and respect the ADA Code of Ethics. (ADA's Code of Ethics can be found in the Appendix.)

Either because of one's prejudice, the need to be confrontational, or misconceptions of mental health counseling, dietetics professionals may hesitate to make referrals to mental health professionals. Learning how and when to make appropriate referrals is part of the ADA Code of Ethics (9) and will be called upon in your expanded role as a nutrition therapist.

Making good referrals means knowing who is in your community. Although this will serve to ultimately help your patients, it also requires up-to-date networking (which was discussed in Chapter 5). Mental health professionals need to know about you, too. They need to know what you do and what to expect when they refer a patient to you. Networking allows you and others to supplement your respective practices.

Massaging Referrals
(Or, How to Get Them Back)

In addition to your therapeutic approach that should convey trust and a desire to help your patients, dietetics professionals still ask: What are the actual mechanics that bring patients back for follow-up appointments? There are some useful techniques to use to encourage follow-up compliance. For answers to some of these questions, see Box 6.3.

If you do your own scheduling, you can set the stage from the first inquiry about your practice. Share your philosophy. Let the prospective client know that there is a process involved in making change . . . and that change takes time. You might share how you structure your sessions. For instance, if you are using the first session as an intake session, it is important to inform the patient of this, so they are not expecting that first session to include in-depth counseling.

Depending on the type of patient you are working with, a technique referred to as previewing may be helpful. Previewing allows prospective patients to know or "preview" some of the topics you hope for them to accomplish. Weight management programs often use previewing by outlining topics that will be covered in subsequent sessions.

BOX 6.3

**WORDS OF WISDOM FROM DIETETICS PROFESSIONALS:
HOW TO GET PATIENTS TO RETURN**

Hilary Warner, MPH, RD, Nutrition Works: "When I schedule the initial appointment, I tell clients that the first appointment is mostly assessment and that the most useful information will be forthcoming. Then I send them an e-mail that includes the following: "The first session is largely devoted to sharing and collecting information—it sets the stage for follow-up visits in which you will really get the nuts and bolts needed to implement the changes necessary for meeting your goals.""

Nancy Clark, MS, RD: "I've found the best way to increase follow-ups is to have people buy a package of three one-hour visits that's less expensive than the three single hours would be. They pay at the end of the first visit when they are inspired."

Andrea Chernus, MS, RD, CDN: "I let the patient know what will happen during the session right at the beginning—i.e. they give me a diet recall, I do a 'nutrition education' piece, and then we set a few goals to work on. I tell them it's taken them ___ years to develop their eating style. One visit with me doesn't automatically erase all their habits."

If you choose to outline goals with your patients, make sure that you break the goals down into achievable "baby steps." It is in a dietitian's nature, as a caregiver and a teacher, to provide patients with as much information as time allows. As a result, the patient may leave a session suffering from information overload. This technique backfires, because it does not allow patients to break the information down into a usable form. Instead, practice providing information in small manageable messages or "sound bites." Patients are much more likely to return if they feel they are making progress. They are also much less likely to feel overwhelmed.

You might find it useful to enter into a contract with a patient, outlining what you both hope to accomplish. This type of previewing encourages follow-up, because the patient has a clear sense of what will be covered in subsequent sessions. When setting up a plan with your patients, be prepared to modify it on the basis of their needs and readiness to use the information.

Learn how and when to end sessions. Sometimes a patient will have more to discuss than time allows in that session. If a patient brings up a topic as the session is ending, acknowledge the importance of the topic and let them know you will be happy to discuss it at the next appointment. Although the patient may feel unsatisfied, it is important that the patient understands and respects your need to adhere to a schedule. Be sure to explain to the patient your desire and intention to answer the questions, allowing the time they warrant. Patients will appreciate your ability to manage your time.

To encourage a patient to return for a follow-up session, close the session with an open-ended question: "When would you like your next appointment" as opposed to "Do you want to come back for follow-up" (11). Be sure you allow time at the end of a session to schedule the follow-up appointment, rather than asking the patient to call you.

Some dietitians find it helpful to provide patients with a written form or card at the end of the session, indicating the follow-up appointment date and time. For an example of a follow-up card, refer to Figure 6.1 on page 144. If you employ a receptionist, you may want to have a policy where he/she places a follow-up call or sends a reminder via e-mail. For an example of a reminder card, see Figure 6.2 on page 144. In one study, patients who received a reminder postcard, telephone call, or detailed information provided in a behavioral contract were more likely to return for follow-up (11).

Some practitioners have found that bundling sessions and giving patients discounts for multiple sessions encourages follow-up. If you use this technique, it is advisable to require payment up front. By using this technique to encourage follow-up, you are also giving patients a "preview" of topics that may be covered in subsequent sessions. Patients may focus on the need to cover specific topics in the sequence that best meets their needs. This ensures that the goals of the sessions are the patient's goals, not the dietitian's goals for the patient.

FIGURE 6.1

Follow-up card.

Jane Doe, MS, RD
Registered Dietitian
555 Fictitious Street
Chicago, Illinois 55555
(555) 555-5555

Mon. _____ AT _____
Tue. _____ AT _____
Wed. _____AT _____
Thu. _____ AT _____
Fri. _____ AT _____

FIGURE 6.2

Reminder card.

You've been missed . . .

Your last nutrition appointment was _____

Please call or email the office to schedule your next appointment.

Jane Doe, MS, RD
(555) 555-5555
email@net.net

Selling Nutrition Therapy

The success of your practice depends on you . . . and how well you can sell yourself. If you are going to sell yourself as a nutrition therapist, referral sources and prospective clients must be aware of your approach, especially if they schedule an appointment with a preconceived idea of what you will do as a dietetics professional. For instance, if a patient has been referred to you because she eats a limited diet and her referring physician and the patient (and family) would like her to eat a more varied diet, the referral sources must be aware that the session will not be an instruction on the foods that need to be added to make a more nutritious diet. Instead, the subsequent sessions will explore why those foods are eliminated and look for ways to motivate the patient to include what it is she has been eliminating. For further information, refer to the case study found in Box 6.4.

BOX 6.4

CASE STUDY OF D.J.

D.J., a fourteen-year-old girl, was referred for nutrition counseling because she was a "picky eater." Her parents were frustrated with her limited food choices and thought a nutrition consultation to "tell her what to eat" was in order. In the first visit, an intake session without D.J. present, the nutrition therapist explained to the parents that she would first need to establish a relationship with the daughter they described as "sassy," to determine why she didn't eat certain foods, before instructing her about what she needed to eat.

D.J. was extremely thin, had not yet started menstruating, and had always been a picky eater. She informed the nutrition therapist that she "knew all about the food pyramid," so the session would probably be a waste of time. As her relationship with food was explored, it was clear that she had been a restrictor since she was 8, because she was afraid of becoming fat. Upon further evaluation, she met the diagnostic criteria for eating disorder, not otherwise specified.

A referral to a family therapist, a pediatrician skilled in working with adolescents, and subsequent sessions with the nutrition therapist uncovered the struggles she was having with food. She is now a healthy, recovered, 21-year-old college student who has a normal weight and eats a wide variety of foods. Had the nutrition therapist merely instructed her in one visit by telling her what was necessary for her to eat, the eating disorder would not have been diagnosed at that point.

Physicians, who are also trained in the medical model, need to be educated about your philosophy, style, and broader therapeutic approach. They may refer their patients to you, expecting that you will "teach" them a prescribed diet. Although you may do this ultimately, there are many steps in between. Since patients may not initially lose weight, reduce their blood pressure, or have greater control over their diabetes, it is important that referring physicians understand your practice. Goals for their patients may not be immediate or measurable in the conventional way. For further information, refer to Box 6.5.

Patients may take small steps toward resolving issues that have kept them from attaining long-term dietary compliance. It may take time for them to reach their ultimate goals. That goal in the end may be different from what the physician originally thought. For instance, a healthier lifestyle without dieting may be a more appropriate goal for a chronic dieter who is depressed. If the physician is using weight loss to assess progress, he/she may need to appreciate the much larger goals you have helped the patient achieve.

Nutrition therapy may be hardest to sell to managed care providers. Managed care visits are most often arranged with a predetermined number of visits. You may be able to impart dietary advice with this arrangement, but you may never see real change unless your patient can communicate the need to have additional visits with you. The reality is, managed care as it stands today may not be conducive to nutrition therapy.

BOX 6.5

CASE STUDY OF S.D.: COMMUNICATING NUTRITION THERAPY TO PHYSICIANS

S.D. was referred for nutrition counseling for hypertension and obesity by his physician. During the intake visit, the nutrition therapist learned that S.D. had recently lost his job, was forced to move back with his family, and was overeating in response to the stress he was feeling. S.D. wanted to improve his diet, lose weight, and begin exercising. However, the nutrition therapist and the patient agreed that his precious health care dollars would be better spent working with a therapist at this point, to help him deal with the other stresses in his life.

The nutrition therapist communicated this to the referring physician, who at first was disappointed that his patient would not be tackling his obvious nutrition problems. After the nutrition therapist explained the overall goals to the physician, he had more realistic expectations for his patient and agreed to monitor his weight and blood pressure. He also agreed to provide encouragement to the patient to work through his personal problems and then to return for nutrition therapy.

If your practice is going to largely be sourced by referrals from managed care health plans, your financial success may depend on high volume. You may need to see many patients for brief visits, and your number of visits with patients may be limited. Your role as a nutrition therapist may be compromised. Your role may need to be more of the traditional model of nutrition educator. This is a need that must be filled in private practice, too. Ideally, you will be able to help those patients and assist them in lobbying their insurance plans to allow the necessary number of visits with you to achieve the identified nutrition goals.

Staying in Business: A Summary

A flourishing private practice may require a change in the traditional approach to dietetics. To encourage follow-up visits, you must position yourself as a nutrition therapist. Successful patients are your best form of advertising. Success will be defined in many ways, but one absolute measure will be whether patients feel satisfied. It may also be necessary to educate referral sources, as well as patients, on more acceptable measures of success.

Keep the following key points in mind:

- Staying in business means growing a practice where repeat business, or follow-up sessions, is a reality.
- Learning how to transition your approach to a counseling style more appropriate for long-term relationships will help you become more successful with your patients.
- Through course work, individual work, and specialized training, you will gradually become more comfortable with your role of nutrition therapist. There are numerous resources available to the dietetics professional, but implementing counseling techniques into your practice is the most useful way to make the transition.
- Communicating your approach to your referral sources and your potential patients is necessary.
- Techniques exist to improve follow-up compliance.

References

1. Maillet J. Dietetics in 2017: what does the future hold? *J Am Diet Assoc.* 2002;102:1404–1406.
2. Reiff D, Reiff K. *Eating Disorders: Nutrition Therapy in the Recovery Process.* Gaithersburg, Md: Aspen Publishers; 1992.

3. Licavoli L. Dietetics goes into therapy. *J Am Diet Assoc.* 1995;95:751–752.

4. Rosal M, Ebbeling C, Lofgren I, Ockene J, Ockene I, Hebert J. Facilitating dietary change: the patient-centered counseling model. *J Am Diet Assoc.* 2001;101:332–341.

5. Coste-Saloff C, Hamburg P, Herzog D. Nutrition and psychotherapy: collaborative treatment of patients with eating disorders. *Bull Menninger Clin.* 1993;57:504–516.

6. McCaffree J. Client satisfaction: turning referrals into regulars. *J Am Diet Assoc.* 2002;102:340–341.

7. Sports Cardiovascular and Wellness Nutritionists. Career tip sheet series: disordered eating. Available at: http://www.scandpg.org/page.asp?id=career_disordered_eating. Accessed March 6, 2004.

8. Kellogg M. Counseling tips for nutrition therapists: the role of supervision. [E-Newsletter]. July 12, 2003. Available at: http://www.mollykellogg.com/Tip%20#%2011%20%20%20The%20Role%20of%20Supervision. Accessed March 6, 2004.

9. American Dietetic Association. Code of ethics for the profession of dietetics. *J Am Diet Assoc.* 1999;99:109–113.

10. American Dietetic Association. Standards of professional practice. *J Am Diet Assoc.* 1998:98:83–85.

11. Myers E, Heffner S. Strategies for improving follow-up client appointment-keeping compliance. *J Am Diet Assoc.* 2001;101:935–939.

Chapter 7

A Brave New World: Putting Technology to Work in Your Practice

The twenty-first century is here. In order to compete in today's market, regardless of the type of business you plan to start, you have to change with the times. Although you do not need to run out and purchase the latest and greatest gadget the minute it appears on the market, you do need to be aware of new technology and assess its usefulness to you.

Technology can save hours of time if you choose the right tools. It can also become costly if you make mistakes in your purchasing. Some equipment is absolutely necessary for running a successful business; some is optional. Purchase the essentials immediately, and purchase nonessential items as your budget allows.

The Essentials

You must have a computer to do business. If you are not computer savvy and do not plan to add that to your list of skills, now is the time to forge a relationship with a good computer consultant or an information technologies (IT) specialist. A computer consultant or IT specialist is someone who plans, develops, operates, maintains, and evaluates computer hardware, software, and telecommunications. He/she can be an invaluable resource to your business. Paying a specialist the hourly rate can save you time and money in the long run.

To locate a good consultant, ask other business owners for recommendations. Look for someone who is used to dealing with small businesses, rather than large companies with huge networks. Get references and check them carefully. Ask how they bill and whether they are available after hours. If so, do rates increase for after-hour calls? Can they help you determine what hardware and software you need? Can they help you get connected by recommending the appropriate Internet option? Finally, can they set it all up? (1)

If your family shares a computer, consider investing in one that is strictly for your business use. You want to have access to the computer at all times, so that you can work when someone else in the house is using the computer.

If the thought of purchasing a computer overwhelms you, the next section will review some basics. Enlist the help of your new IT consultant, rather than relying on the salespeople at the computer store, to guide you through this process.

Computer Hardware

Your first decision to make is whether to purchase a laptop computer or a desktop computer. If you will be traveling to different locations, giving presentations, or want round-the-clock access to your files, you will need a laptop. If you see patients in a location other than your main office, bringing a laptop will allow you to enter your new patient information, as well as process fees and collections immediately after each visit. You can also work on other projects if you have a gap in your schedule, a cancellation, or a no-show. A laptop provides you with the freedom to do your work when and where you wish.

If you are accustomed to using a desktop computer, you may have a hard time adjusting to a laptop. The screen and keyboard may be smaller, and some people find the laptop or built-in mouse hard to use. To accommodate these less-than-ideal conditions, you can set up a docking station in your home office, which will allow you to connect your laptop to a standard monitor, keyboard, and mouse. You can also bring along an external mouse, which you can easily plug directly into your laptop.

If you do not travel and basically have one office in which you do everything, then a traditional desktop system should meet your needs (2). In this case, your basic hardware will include a monitor, a mouse, a keyboard, and a CPU (central processing unit). Although all these components can be bought separately, generally it is easiest to purchase a package that contains all of them. Later, you can determine which of these components you prefer to upgrade.

MONITORS

Monitors come in CRT (cathode-ray tube), LCD (liquid crystal display) plasma, touch screen, TV, and cable-ready (1). As of this writing, the LCD and plasma screens are state-of-the-art and are priced considerably higher. Seventeen inches (measured diagonally) is generally considered the standard size for a monitor.

CPU

The CPU provides the speed for the computer. It is also referred to as the microprocessor. For everyday word processing, spreadsheets, and e-mail, 2.66 ghz is sufficient processor speed (3). When you see the words "Intel inside" printed on your computer, that refers to the CPU (1). You can also purchase a wireless mouse and keyboard, which will decrease the number of wires coming out of your computer.

MEMORY

Within the CPU is the machine's random access memory (RAM). RAM is measured in megabytes. Purchase as much memory as you can afford. Memory enables you to run several programs at once. Most moderately priced computers come with 256 MB of RAM, but for efficiency and speed it is recommended that you have a minimum of 512 MB (3).

PRINTER

There are several options for printers, and the prices range widely. Laser printers provide permanent prints and will cost considerably more than inkjet printers. However, most inkjet printers require costly ink replacement cartridges. Factoring this in, if you plan to print a lot, a laser printer can save money because the cost per page is considerably less than for an inkjet printer (4). If you think you will be printing a lot, consider investing in a black-and-white laser printer. A color laser printer is your most expensive option. Businesses that work with graphic arts tend to invest in laser printers. For most small businesses, a good-quality color inkjet printer will be sufficient.

MODEM

A modem is used for Internet access, electronic faxes, and e-mail. You need to choose between a "dial-up" modem, which uses a standard telephone line for Internet access; a DSL line, which also uses a telephone line but does not tie up your telephone; and a cable modem, which is accessed through a separate cable, usually installed by your cable television provider. DSL and cable modems are for broadband Internet. They require special connections and provide much faster service than dial-up. However, the monthly fees are higher than those of telephone lines. For most businesses, broadband is worth the extra investment because it saves time.

COMPACT DISK RECORDER

A compact disk (CD) recorder, sometimes referred to as a CD burner, allows you to provide clients or colleagues with large files electronically. It also is an excellent way to back up your files. Most new computers come with an internal CD burner. If you have a computer without one, you can also buy an external CD burner.

DVD RECORDER

A DVD recorder, sometimes referred to as a DVD burner, is similar to a CD recorder but holds about six times as much data. You will also pay more for one. Some new computers are built with internal DVD burners.

MISCELLANEOUS HARDWARE

Other hardware that you may want to consider adding to your package includes the following:

- *Multipurpose scanner, fax machine, copier, printer.* The multipurpose scanner, fax machine, copier, printer is sometimes referred to as an "all-in-one." The all-in-one can save space by taking the place of several pieces of equipment. It provides general coverage for business usage, but you can't use it for high-volume copying or printing. This might be a good option for the practitioner who does not have much office space.
- *Removable media storage device.* Removable storage devices, such as the Zip drive, used to be quite popular, but they have been largely replaced by removable CD or DVD drives. A removable storage device allows larger quantities of data to be written onto the disks. There are 100-Mb and 250-Mb disks available. Although these devices are useful for transferring large files and for system backups, the CD recorder or DVD recorder is a much better option for a private practice with a limited budget.
- *Digital camera.* If you plan to do work for presentations, a digital camera may be an important accessory. Digital pictures can be used to add

great visuals to PowerPoint presentations. There are a wide variety of digital cameras available, and the prices vary. Research these carefully, or consult with your IT consultant, before purchasing.

As a general rule, when purchasing hardware, it is best to avoid the least expensive equipment. However, top of the line is rarely necessary.

Purchase a computer with a warranty from a reputable and reliable store. If being without your computer will put you out of business, it is recommended that you purchase a service contract as an "insurance policy." This will allow for continued productivity in the event that your computer malfunctions and needs repair. Refer to Box 7.1 for more technology tips.

BOX 7.1

BYTES OF WISDOM, BY BRUCE MALIKEN, UP AND RUNNING COMPUTER SERVICES, LLC

- When purchasing your computer, be wary of the one-person operation. Who will mind the store when that person is away?

- Choose high-speed Internet—cable or DSL. Telephone dial-up is OK if you are using the Internet only for e-mail.

- When selecting memory, get a minimum of 512 megabytes of RAM, but purchase as much as you can afford.

- You can obtain a free e-mail account through the following ISPs: yahoo.com, myway.com, hotmail.com.

- Do not let your kids load video games onto your business computer. The video and audio portions of some programs are so resource-intensive that they could be potentially damaging to your office software.

- Keep all software and paraphernalia (instruction booklets, disks, etc.) organized in one place. If you need repair or upgrades, it is much easier to accomplish.

- Store your computer equipment in a safe, secure, clean place.

Computer Software

The computer software you need to consider falls under a few categories. You will need office management software, antivirus software, and probably nutrient analysis software. If you have a very specialized business, you may look at niche software (5).

OFFICE MANAGEMENT SOFTWARE

When you purchase a computer package, it usually comes with an office software package. Typically, this includes a word processing program and one or two other programs, such as a spreadsheet application and a presentation program. A good accounting software package is an asset to your business and will save you valuable time. You can keep track of all your financial data and client billing with the right program. Chapter 5 reviews the basics of choosing accounting software.

You can also use your computer's software to enhance your practice and streamline your work in numerous ways. Software packages can handle all your administrative tasks. For most small businesses, there are many good programs to handle accounting and billing. For example, it is possible to keep records of all new patients and to track how each patient was referred to you. If you wanted to determine who your top referral sources were, you could easily access that information. Box 7.2 offers an example of practice management software in use.

You can create assessment forms using your word processing program. By creating templates as your original, you can make as many copies as you need. Another option is to enter the assessment data right into the form, and save that form as part of the patient's computerized chart. A similar principle can be applied to reports for referral sources. Develop a template, and use it each time you need to send a report. Fill in the blanks, and save one copy as part of the patient's chart. Print one copy to send to the referral source (5).

You can also create unique educational materials using your word processing program and some creativity. Use clip art to jazz them up and maintain the patient's interest (5).

If creating these forms does not appeal to you, or you simply do not have the time, there are a few other options. You can purchase the forms as hard copies and scan them into your computer (provided you have a scanner). This allows you to print them out as needed. You can also purchase forms on disk. Chapter 9 lists resources where you can find these products. You can also hire a tech-savvy dietitian to help you.

BOX 7.2

HOW ONE RD USES COMPUTER SOFTWARE FOR PRACTICE MANAGEMENT

Carolyn Bell, RD, of Nutrition and Diet Services, LLC, uses the ACT! software program to streamline her practice. When she first began with the program, she hired a consultant for approximately four hours to come in and teach her and her associates how to navigate and customize the program for their practice's services.

They use the software to

- Schedule appointments

- E-mail clients

- Send personalized letters to clients and physicians

- Track referrals

- Track where their clients are coming from (geographically)

- Track why clients came to them

- Code their appointments

The software is crucial to their day-to-day operations. They created their own codes to enhance their use. The codes they created help them identify the referral source for each new patient, what needs to be done at the initial visit, and how much time to allow.

ANTIVIRUS SOFTWARE

An antivirus package is essential to your private practice, especially if you are using the Internet. Spend the money to add this to your system. You can get a good antivirus program that also comes with a firewall. Firewalls monitor "traffic" along the border between your computer and the Internet. The firewall prevents "hackers"—people who intentionally try to exploit your computer to intercept information—from accessing your computer. These two programs should protect your computer from damaging outside influences. Some companies sell good bundle packages. After installing the software, it is critical to download your antivirus updates regularly and set your computer to do automatic virus definition updates and system scans (6).

NUTRIENT ANALYSIS SOFTWARE

Some dietetics professionals remember having to perform nutrient calculations by hand. Analyzing a recipe or someone's 3-day food diary was tedious and time-consuming work. Enter nutrient analysis software. Today's programs have streamlined the work of dietetics professionals, allowing them to spend more time with their patients or to market their programs and practices.

Nutrient analysis software is a valuable addition to any dietetic practice. Many packages are available. Check the resources in Chapter 9 for a list of some options. If you want to investigate a number of programs and actually try them out, download trial versions and/or plan to attend ADA's Food and Nutrition Conference and Expo (FNCE), where many of the companies exhibit their products.

Before you purchase nutrition software, evaluate your needs. Decide what you need your software to do. Make a list of essential features and rate them in importance. Depending on your practice setting and your patient population, your needs may vary. Before you purchase, refer to Box 7.3 for a list of questions to ask about each program (7,8).

BOX 7.3

EVALUATING NUTRITION SOFTWARE: QUESTIONS TO ASK

- How reliable is the nutrient database?

- Can you manipulate data in various ways—i.e., subtract an ingredient from a recipe?

- Can you track numerous patients simultaneously?

- Can you add food items to the database?

- How easy is it to find a food from the database?

- Can you plan meals at various calorie levels with various nutrient distributions?

- What type of printouts can you get?

- Can you customize printouts?

- Are updates free?

- Will software be used by more than one person? Is that authorized?

- Does software need to be available in more than one location?

- Is technical support provided?

Source: Data are from Fiske H. 2002 nutrition software review. *Today's Dietitian.* 2002;4:22–28 and Prestwood E. Nutrition software: 101 questions to ask before you buy. Available at: http://www.dietsoftware.com/101.html. Accessed December 15, 2003.

Nutrition analysis software can aid in clinical assessment. It can help you determine the adequacy of a patient's diet and highlight specific deficiencies. In private practice, this software can be a powerful teaching tool. Providing analysis to your patient helps them visualize their nutrition goals. The printouts provide tangible evidence and feedback, which help them stay focused.

Providing nutrient analysis to your patients is a value-added service. It takes additional time to analyze a patient's diet. Determine whether you want to provide that service to your patients as an additional benefit. As an alternative, you may want to charge for the service separately, as a way to generate further revenue. It can be a great marketing tool. Some dietetics professionals offer nutrient analysis as a stand-alone service.

If you have a specific need in your practice that a general nutrient analysis software package does not meet, consider purchasing niche software. For example, if you see many diabetic patients, you may want to purchase a specialized program that is geared toward that patient population. There are programs that assist you in teaching your patient about diabetic nutrition. One specialized program explains diabetic meal planning principles and enables the patient to plan sample meals. It also allows you to enter the patient's needs and help them make correct food choices (5).

Using the Internet

Using the Internet in your practice can be quite an asset. Most practitioners cannot function without it. The myriad opportunities that exist, in both promotion and research, have opened up many doors for dietetics professionals.

E-mail

E-mail has greatly increased productivity. In many cases, e-mail has replaced the telephone call. Dietetics professionals use e-mail to communicate with business associates regarding business issues or scheduling meetings. They may communicate with other health care professionals regarding a particular patient.

Some dietetics professionals have patients e-mail their daily food records. "New patient information" can be sent via e-mail, including directions, office policies, information about your practice, and any forms that need to be filled out. They can be sent as an attachment before your first visit with a new patient.

Some dietetics professionals provide online counseling. Others lead online counseling groups. Consult with your malpractice insurance carrier to verify your coverage for online counseling. Your insurance carrier may also be able to advise you regarding licensing issues. The question has been raised as to whether a dietetics professional must be licensed in all of the states in which she provides patient counseling.

Discussing patients with other health care providers, communicating with patients via e-mail, and providing online counseling are all considered Protected Health Information (PHI) under Health Insurance Portability and Accountability Act (HIPAA) guidelines. HIPAA regulations do not prohibit the use of e-mail; however, the law requires that individuals and organizations take steps to decrease or eliminate the risk of unauthorized interception of transmissions or the receipt of information by unauthorized individuals.

Although there is no specific recommended method for preventing unauthorized reception of information, providers use various techniques, including the following:

- Closed networks
- Virtual private networks
- Encryption services

For more detailed information on this subject, ZixCorp provides an excellent resource at its Web site (http://www.zixcorp.com/hipaa/faq.php).

For those discussing particular patients via e-mail, it is also recommended that a confidentiality notice be placed at the bottom of the e-mail. See Chapter 3 for a sample notice.

Listservs and Electronic Mailing Lists

Electronic mailing lists and listservs are wonderful free tools for dietetics professionals. A listserv is a forum for discussion via e-mail. You can "subscribe" to listservs that pertain to your area of interest. When you send an e-mail message to a listserv, everyone who is subscribed receives the e-mail (9). Dietetics professionals use listservs to obtain clinical and business advice from colleagues across the country, announce consulting positions, and locate referrals for their patients who are moving.

The ADA has a general listserv open to all members. Most of the dietetic practice groups (DPGs) also have listservs, which are more specialized by area of practice. Even within the DPGs, listservs exist among subgroups. For example, the Nutrition Entrepreneurs DPG has a general listserv as well as specific listservs for authors, speakers, Internet, and private practice. Participating in the DPG listservs requires membership in that DPG.

E-mail can also be used as a marketing tool. Collect e-mail addresses from your patients, and e-mail them the "recipe of the month" or the "nutrition tip of the month." Make sure you have permission, however. You do not want to be the source of unwanted mail.

The World Wide Web As Research and Marketing Tool

Staying current is essential in private practice. Your patients will want your opinion of the latest diet or today's news about food safety. To stay current, you can subscribe online to major newspapers, such as *The New York Times, The Wall Street Journal,* or *The Washington Post.*

You can also use search engines to look up content on just about any topic. A search engine is a tool that enables users to locate information on the World Wide Web. Users enter keywords to locate Web sites containing the information they seek. This will allow you to see what the public is reading. Box 7.4 provides a listing of search engines you can use to find almost anything (10). Carefully evaluate the information you find via these search engines. It may not always be credible.

When it comes to research about food and nutrition, it is important to consult credible Web sites. Box 7.5 (see page 160) lists sites that ADA has recommended to provide reliable information (11). Additionally, the Web sites listed in Chapter 9 provide reliable nutrition information; most of them are geared for the general public.

You can access educational materials online, but be aware of legal rules regarding the distribution of such documents to patients. Materials published by the U.S. government are generally part of the public domain and usually can be distributed without asking permission. Other material on the Internet is copyrighted. Many Web sites allow you to reprint copyrighted documents

---

BOX 7.4

POPULAR SEARCH ENGINES

- Google: http://www.google.com

- Ask Jeeves: http://www.ask.com

- Hotbot: http://www.hotbot.com

- Yahoo: http://www.yahoo.com

- Exactseek: http://www.exactseek.com

- Netscape Search: http://www.netscape.com

Source: Used with permission from The Small Business Advisor. Available at: http://www.isquare.com.

BOX 7.5
WEB SITES THAT ADA TRUSTS

- PubMed: http://www.ncbi.nlm.nih.gov/PubMed

- National Center for Health Statistics: http://www.cdc.gov.nchs

- Gateway to Government Food Safety Information: http://www.foodsafety.gov

- Food and Nutrition Information Center: http://www.nal.usda.gov/fnic/index.html

- MEDLINEplus: http://www.medlineplus.gov

- Office of Dietary Supplements: http://ods.od.nih.gov/index.aspx

- Food and Drug Administration Food Labeling and Nutrition: http://www.cfsan.fda.gov/label.html

- Center for Nutrition Policy and Promotion: http://www.usda.gov/cnpp

- Journal of the American Dietetic Association: http://www.adajournal.org

- USDA National Nutrient Database for Standard Reference: http://www.nal.usda.gov/fnic/foodcomp

- National Academy of Sciences Institute of Medicine: http://www.iom.edu

Source: Adapted with permission from American Dietetic Association. Reliable information on the Internet. *ADA Times.* 2003;1:2. Copyright © 2003 American Dietetic Association.

for free if you are using them for educational purposes (5). However, you should always verify that reprints are permitted before you distribute materials. You may need a signed release from the copyright holder; some copyright holders will charge a fee for use. Another option is to direct your patients to some of the sites you deem appropriate and accurate.

Use the Web as a marketing tool. Subscribe to online referral listings. ADA's Nationwide Nutrition Network provides a referral listing at no charge to members. Be sure to check other health associations, such as the American Diabetes Association, for opportunities to list your practice.

Many of these referral listings allow you to list your e-mail address for contact information. Once you do, be prepared for inquiries via e-mail about your services. You may find it beneficial to save some marketing materials, such as your bio and information about your practice, as electronic documents. You can then send them to potential patients as you receive e-mail requests.

Web Site for Your Practice

In this Internet-savvy age, dietetics professionals may jump to the conclusion that they need a Web site to be credible. Although many dietetics professionals have developed Web sites, developing and maintaining a Web site can be costly and time consuming.

Web sites serve several purposes for the dietetics professional. They can be used to provide prospective clients with information about your practice in the same way a printed brochure might be used. They can be used in an interactive way, to communicate with clients and potential clients. They can also be used to sell products (12,13).

If you have the time, interest, and inclination, you can develop your own Web site. Alternatively, you can hire a Web site designer to develop it for you. Before you choose a designer, look at other sites he/she has created. See if they appeal to you. Even if you hire a designer, you must be involved at every step of the way. Once it is designed, you need to host it or hire someone to host and maintain it. Again, all these processes are costly or will require your time.

Before you create your Web site, think about how you want to use it, whether you have the time and skill to develop it, and how much time you are willing to devote to it. Just having a presence on the Web is not the reason for having a Web site, unless you see it as an efficient or effective way to communicate with your clients. The resources mentioned in Chapter 9 will be useful to consult before designing your own site or selecting a Web site designer.

Personal Digital Assistants

Today, 30% of dietitians use personal digital assistants (PDAs) in their practice, and 35% are considering buying one (14). A PDA is an electronic organizer and minicomputer (15). PDAs contain software programs, offer a built-in calculator, have the ability to download information from the Web, and send e-mail (15).

Although some dietetics professionals use their PDAs primarily for standard functions, such as address book, scheduling, to-do lists, and expense reports, their usefulness in the private practice setting extends well beyond these areas. Here are some ways you can use your PDA to further enhance your practice (15,16):

- Enter formulas to perform calculations, such as calorie requirements, body mass index (BMI), resting metabolic rate (RMR), and so on.
- Download resources, such as the *Physician's Desk Reference,* nutrient analyses, or sources of vitamins and minerals. Have all your resources right at your fingertips.
- Store patient information (be sure to enter a password so no one else can access your PDA).
- Coordinate with patients—send them information or have them keep daily food logs on their PDAs, if they have one, too.

Add a PDA to the growing list of technology you can't live without. This small piece of equipment, the size of a calculator, can take the place of several pieces of equipment. Refer to Box 7.6 for more on this topic (16).

BOX 7.6

TOP TEN REASONS FOR NUTRITION PROFESSIONALS TO OWN A PDA

---

10. Provide more comprehensive patient care . . . faster.

9. Convert milliequivalents to milligrams without looking for your conversion table.

8. When you want to check for drug-nutrient interactions, you can look it up instantly and inconspicuously.

7. When you're waiting for the train or plane, or in line at the store, update all your business expenses . . . or better yet, play solitaire!

6. Do calorie needs, protein needs, adjusted weight, ideal weight, etc., in seconds.

5. Never forget another appointment, birthday, or anniversary—let your alarm remind you.

4. Look up the fat content of an avocado or the calcium content of tofu in less than 10 seconds.

3. When a doctor asks you for your business card, beam it instantly. Heck, beam her your whole resume.

2. Know that your to-do list, shopping list, and holiday gift list are a tap away, and be able to check them off when they're done.

1. Empty your lab coat, handbag, computer bag, briefcase, or backpack of all those books and papers. You can have the same information and more in your PDA!

Source: Reprinted with permission from Aronson D. Top 10 Reasons for Nutrition Professionals to Own a PDA. Available at: http://www.pdaRD.com. Accessed January 10, 2004.

Nutrition Assessment Tools

Body Fat Analyzers

Body fat analyzers can be very helpful to dietetics professionals in private practice. They allow patients and practitioners to measure progress in ways other than the scale. Patients ask dietetics professionals to analyze their body fat, and it can be expected as part of the nutrition assessment. Sports nutritionists find them to be a useful tool, as do eating disorder and weight management professionals.

You need to first decide whether it makes sense to provide body fat analysis to your patients. If so, decide whether to provide it at no charge or to use it as a value-added service. Some dietetics professionals charge an additional fee for the service, as a way of recouping the expense of the equipment.

There are many handheld body fat analyzers on the market. It is important to assess their reliability and accuracy before you purchase one. Evaluate their accuracy with different patient populations—for example, very low body fat individuals with anorexia. Ask other professionals what they recommend, and do your own research. Select a technology that works best for your practice and your patients.

Metabolic Testing

Another gadget that can complement your practice is a calorimeter. This tool measures RMR using indirect calorimetry. It is a useful tool for the dietetics professional working with athletes, chronic dieters, or eating-disordered patients, and it can add value to your practice. As with body fat analyzers, you should research the options, ask for recommendations, and select the brand that fits your practice and your patient population.

A Brave New World: A Summary

Depending on your interest level, the opportunities you have had, and maybe even your age, you may or may not be using technology to your best advantage. If the task of putting technology to work for you is daunting, find someone who can assist you with that task. Find a mentor with expertise in technology and offer to assist her with some aspect of her practice. The Nutrition Entrepreneurs DPG has a technology subunit dedicated to helping dietetics professionals advance their technological knowledge and skills. Box 7.7 (see page 164) provides an example of ways in which technology has helped to streamline one dietetics professional's workload.

BOX 7.7

A DAY IN THE LIFE OF A TECH-SAVVY RD

Dina Aronson, MS, RD, a nutrition consultant, author, editor, and speaker, who works from her home office in Medford, MA, depends on technology for her consulting work. The following table summarizes Dina's current projects and how she uses technology to get the job done.

Project	Technology Used
Consulting for a company on the production of a nutrition calculator that will be sold at retail chains across the country. Her job is to help design the product and to set up the food database according to the company's specifications.	Microsoft Access Database; Microsoft Excel; Microsoft Word; Internet/E-mail
Editing, formatting, and marketing a set of nutrition education handouts for a nutrition and corporate wellness company. Creating a CD-Rom to sell with the handouts.	Graphic design and desktop publishing programs (Quark Express, Adobe Acrobat, Adobe Illustrator, Adobe Photoshop); CD burner, Internet/E-mail
Cowriting a book on food allergies.	Online database–driven search engines for research; Internet/E-mail
Preparing a presentation on the topic of Web design for a state association meeting.	Microsoft PowerPoint; Internet/E-mail
Meeting with a client for a nutrition counseling follow-up session.	Palm Pilot (applications that calculate energy and protein needs); nutrition analysis software
Updating her Web sites with "handout of the week" (nutrawiz.com) and "tip of the week" (pdaRD.com).	Web site software; FTP client (program that transfers files to and from the Internet); Internet/E-mail
Ongoing work: checking e-mail, organizing activities, scheduling meetings, prioritizing tasks, paperwork, and billing.	Palm Pilot; Microsoft Outlook; financial management software; Internet/E-mail

Dina notes that technology is a tool that enhances her work, not the foundation of her work. Her expertise as a dietitian is her most valuable skill. For example, for the database consulting work, knowledge of nutrition and foods is imperative in creating a database that best suits the needs of the customer. Dina believes that knowing how to use Microsoft Access gave her an edge in being chosen for the project.

Once you begin to use all your new "toys," you'll be accomplished in no time. With each technological addition, you won't be able to imagine how you ever did without it.

Keep in mind the following key points:

- A computer is essential for managing your business and saving you time.
- If you are not comfortable with technology, consider hiring an IT consultant or a tech-savvy dietitian to assist you.
- You must have office management software and antivirus software. Most private practitioners can use nutrient analysis software. If you are highly specialized, consider niche software.
- Dietetics professionals can use e-mail to communicate with other health professionals, provide patient counseling, and send out "new patient information." They can also stay connected by participating in electronic mailing lists.
- The World Wide Web can be used for monitoring nutrition news, accessing educational materials, and marketing your practice.
- Developing a Web site can be costly and time consuming. Before you create a Web site, analyze the purpose of the site and whether you have the necessary resources to keep it up and running.

References

1. Friedman C, Yorio K. *The Girl's Guide to Starting Your Own Business: Candid Advice, Frank Talk, and True Stories for the Successful Entrepreneur.* New York, NY: HarperCollins; 2003.
2. Obringer L. How setting up a home office works: what hardware do you need? [How Stuff Works Web site]. Available at: http://money.howstuffworks.com/home-office.htm/printable. Accessed December 24, 2003.
3. How to buy a desktop PC [PC World Web site]. Available at: http://www.pcworld.com/howto/bguide/0,guid,14,00.asp. Accessed March 3, 2004.
4. How to buy a printer [PC World Web site]. Available at: http://www.pcworld.com/howto/bguide/0,guid,16,00.asp. Accessed March 3, 2004.
5. Clairmont C. A hard look at software solutions to ease your workload. *Today's Dietitian.* 2001;3:24–27.
6. Aronson D. Preventing computer disasters. *Today's Dietitian.* 2004;6:46–49.
7. Fiske H. 2002 nutrition software review. *Today's Dietitian.* 2002;4:22–28.
8. Prestwood E. Nutrition software: 101 questions to ask before you buy. Available at: http://www.dietsoftware.com/101.html. Accessed December 15, 2003.
9. Aronson D. Make the most out of e-mail. *DBC Dimensions.* Fall 2003:6.

10. Small Business Advisor. Web search sites. Available at: http://www.isquare.com/fhame7.cfm. Accessed December 4, 2003.

11. American Dietetic Association. Where can I find reliable information about food and nutrition? *ADA Times.* 2003;1:1–2.

12. Pangan T, Bednar C. Dietitian business Web sites: a survey of their profitability and how you can make yours profitable. *J Am Diet Assoc.* 2001:101:399–402.

13. Pangan T. Laying down the foundation of a successful Web site. *Ventures: Enterprising News and Ideas for Nutrition Entrepreneurs,* 2003;19:3–4.

14. Aronson D. Tools of the trade: high tech gadgets for dietitians. *Today's Dietitian.* 2003;5:34-36.

15. Aronson D. Personal digital assistants (PDAs): toy or necessity? Available at: http://www.pdaRD.com. Accessed January 10, 2004.

16. Aronson D. Top 10 reasons for nutrition professionals to own a PDA. Available at: http://www.pdaRD.com. Accessed January 10, 2004.

Chapter 8

The Sky's the Limit: Turning Your Experience into Dollars

If you have decided to enter private practice or consulting, you might want to consider exploring other options and opportunities available to you. The sky truly is the limit! Dietetics professionals have exhibited creative ways to use their education and skills that have resulted in opportunities, positions, and, ultimately, money. In this chapter, we will explore various avenues of consulting, not just private practice.

Dietetics professionals across the country have taken the risk and left their jobs to become self-employed. The ADA 2002 Dietetics Compensation and Benefits Survey indicated that 10% of RDs who responded to the survey were self-employed, whereas 11% indicated that they worked in private practice/consultation to individuals or consultation/contract services to organizations. However, 6% of RDs indicated that they were owners or partners in their practice (1). Starting a consulting business or a private practice in the field of dietetics is clearly a viable option for those dietetics professionals willing to take the plunge.

Defining the Word "Consultant"

Throughout this book, the terms "private practice" and "consulting" have been differentiated. The difference is based on what one does in one's business. If you are setting up shop to provide individual nutrition counseling, you are in private practice. For the purposes of this book, all other entrepreneurial endeavors are referred to as consulting.

The Internal Revenue Service (IRS) has a very specific set of criteria that one must meet in order to legally be a consultant for tax purposes. Box 8.1 summarizes the IRS criteria (2).

BOX 8.1

CRITERIA FOR INDEPENDENT CONTRACTOR STATUS

Behavioral Control

An independent contractor decides the following:

- How, when, and where to do the work

- What tools or equipment to use

- What assistants (if any) to hire to help with the work

- Where to purchase supplies and services

- Which methods will be used to perform services (training is not provided)

Financial Control

According to the following criteria, the independent contractor controls business aspects of the work:

- Contractor has a significant investment in the facilities used for the work.

- Contractor is not reimbursed for most expenses.

- Contractor can incur a loss or realize a profit.

Business Relationship

For the independent contractor, the following are true:

- Employee benefits are not provided to the contractor.

- A written contract may indicate independent contractor status.

- An independent contractor usually has a less permanent relationship with a company than an employee would have.

Source: Data are from Internal Revenue Service. *Employer's Supplemental Tax Guide.* Washington, DC: US Department of Treasury; 2004. IRS Publication 15A.

It may be beneficial to work with an accountant or business adviser to determine your status. For the purposes of this chapter, a consultant is defined as someone who is self-employed, who is not an employee of any organization or company, and who is paid to provide a specific service.

Market Trends

Consulting and/or home-based businesses are increasing in numbers, indicating a very popular market trend (1). Whenever there is a downturn in the economy, the numbers of consultants in the marketplace increase. This makes sense, because when one is unemployed in a slow economy, consulting is a viable employment opportunity. In April 2003, the House of Delegates of the American Dietetic Association recognized the importance of the report "Trend Alert," by Roger and Joyce Herman of the Herman Group. The following paragraphs are very significant (3):

> It is a well-known fact that the strongest growth in employment comes from small business, not major corporations. Small businesses form a stable and active sub-economy. Recognized or not, small companies—including "microbusinesses" with just a few employees, are in the vast majority of businesses everywhere.
>
> During the economic slowdown, many people formed small businesses, the majority operating from the owner's home. These new businesses successfully generated income to survive this difficult period. As the economy improves, these micropreneurs will think carefully about whether they want to rejoin the corporate rat race. The increasingly robust economy will provide more opportunities for new business creation.

The RD who has recently lost his or her job at the hospital because of downsizing is in a position to use the same skills to start a private practice. Once in the field of consulting, many professionals find it to be more gratifying than their old role of employee. If you have your own business, you will have a much more flexible schedule. You decide your work hours.

Many people find consulting much more compatible with family life. You are able to take time off for personal reasons. You must, however, be careful not to "abuse" this privilege. If you take too much time off, you cannot meet your clients' needs. Then your career looks more like a hobby.

In addition to the flexibility, many consultants find that they are able to "simplify" their lives. Working from home eliminates the commute each day, allowing more productive time. Regular office hours can be much more flexible than the typical "nine to five," with the potential of earning more money. Some private practitioners hold office hours during evenings and weekends, thus eliminating the need for childcare. This creates a very coveted marketing niche. Some "empty nesters" whose spouses are retired are finding that private practice allows them the flexibility to enjoy those years as well.

Reportedly, consultants generally earn more money than employees. The ADA 2002 Dietetics Compensation and Benefits Survey indicates that "RDs self-employed in private practice or as consultants do markedly better than RDs in others' employ, on average" (1). See Figure 8.1 for more information.

FIGURE 8.1

RD hourly wage by employer status. Reprinted with permission from American Dietetic Association. *2002 Dietetics Compensation and Benefits Survey.* Chicago, Ill: American Dietetic Association; 2003:15.

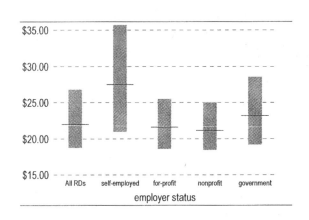

			Percentiles	
	#	25th	50th	75th
All RDs	8,621	$18.75	$22.00	$26.79
Self-employed	796	$21.00	$27.47	$35.69
For-profit	2,591	$18.63	$21.63	$25.50
Nonprofit (other than government)	3,389	$18.46	$21.15	$25.00
Government	1,704	$19.23	$23.20	$28.55

Consulting Opportunities

The various types of consulting for dietetics professionals are endless now. Years ago, most consultant dietitians were either consulting to health care facilities or providing individual patient counseling. This is no longer the case.

Dietetics professionals have taken their skills and expertise and have developed opportunities for themselves that would not have been considered "dietetics" at all. For example, some dietitians are personal trainers, lactation consultants, registered nurses, or professional speakers. Some have dual degrees or certificates or another type of additional training. The goal of this chapter is to provide as many ideas and examples as possible, to enable you to map out your game plan, to branch out, and to supplement your private practice.

As you formulate your ideas, you will probably consider the need to have various arrangements simultaneously. Earning income doing just one type of consulting is quite a challenge. Try your hand at various types of consulting, to figure out what you enjoy and what you do not. What are you best at? What is your forte? You may even combine consulting positions with some that are nonconsulting, particularly if you need to earn extra income or retain some benefits. For example, consider accepting a part-time position as a clinical dietitian in a hospital while you develop your private practice.

In some cases, you may need to provide your services for free. Before you do so, ask yourself, "Is it a marketing opportunity?" This motto is an important mantra to remember.

Private Practice

Although a dietitian in private practice can provide nutrition counseling to groups, he/she primarily provides individual counseling. The ADA dietetic practice group (DPG) Nutrition Entrepreneurs consists of dietitians who not only have their own nutrition counseling practices but also write books, design nutrition products, and perform other nutrition-related jobs, which will be detailed later in this chapter. Nutrition Entrepreneurs is the DPG to join if you need mentoring and help in establishing your private practice. Members receive a quarterly newsletter, *Ventures,* and the DPG offers numerous services to its members to support the entrepreneur. Further information on this resource can be found at the DPG's Web site (http://www.nutritionentrepreneurs.org).

Many dietetics professionals across the country have left their jobs and started their own nutrition counseling practices. The benefits of controlling their own schedules, potentially making more money and doing things "their way" make this change very appealing. Many dietetics professionals mention that they are ready for a change or are just tired of working for someone else.

For many, individual counseling is their primary source of income. They spend most of their working time providing individual or group nutrition counseling for a fee. This is a particularly easy transition for clinical dietitians who have been providing nutrition education to their patients in the hospital setting. They have the experience in counseling and they often have the contacts.

Many practitioners find that they need to diversify once they have established their private practices. Burnout is one reason for diversification. Providing one-on-one counseling 4 to 5 days per week does have the potential to create burnout in the counselor. It is important to schedule breaks frequently. The more days per week one is counseling, the more frequently he/she should consider scheduling a vacation or mental health day, even if that day is just devoted to catching up on paperwork or cleaning out the office.

Private practice can be isolating. Your day is spent helping others and listening to others' problems, and depending on your office situation, you may have little interaction with other professionals. It is important to stay connected to other professionals. Make sure to do the following:

- Join professional organizations
- Attend conferences
- Schedule lunch with colleagues
- Talk on the phone with colleagues
- Take advantage of the various electronic mailing lists and chats available through ADA's DPGs

Another reason for diversification is to increase income. Most dietitians in private practice find that diversification just happens. Once established in private practice, they begin to receive calls for other types of nutrition-related jobs.

When you are seeing patients by the hour and therefore billing by the hour, there are only so many hours you can bill. When you don't see patients, you don't make money, so it is tempting to keep squeezing more patients in. A psychotherapist considers a full-time workweek 25 to 30 patient-hours per week, thus allowing time in the remainder of the "typical" 40-hour week for paperwork, telephone calls, professional interaction, and down time.

The demand for nutrition professionals in private practice is growing. Physicians now regularly refer their patients to RDs for nutrition counseling. Individuals also seek nutrition counseling without physician referrals. Kids today find it "cool" to talk about who their nutritionist is! With the acceptance of medical nutrition therapy being reimbursable by Medicare and other insurance for certain medical conditions, the need for private practitioners is increasing. In some areas of the United States, there seems to be a shortage of dietetics practitioners. The established, well-known practitioners have waiting lists. If you look for an RD on the American Dietetic Association's Nationwide Referral Network, in some areas of the country you draw a blank. This indicates that the demand is greater than the supply, so there is quite a market for private practitioners across the country.

Consulting for Health Care Facilities

Many types of facilities, such as nursing homes, dialysis centers, group homes, hospices, HMOs, day treatment hospitals, and certain types of rehabilitation facilities, do not have the budget to pay a registered dietitian's salary on a full-time basis. However, regulations do require the services of an RD, for them to maintain their licenses.

In this type of arrangement, the registered dietitian is employed under contract to provide nutrition consultation to acute-care and long-term-care facilities, health agencies, home-care companies, and even the foodservice industry. Hence, an entire category of consulting opportunities—consulting for health care facilities—is open to the dietitian.

Many dietetics professionals have successful consulting businesses in which they consult to numerous facilities, also referred to as "accounts." Often, state regulations in certain health care facilities require an RD's services for a minimum number of hours each month. Of course, this varies from state to state, but if you are interested in pursuing this type of consulting, it would be beneficial to check the regulations in your state.

There are many resources available for a dietitian who wants to begin to consult to health care facilities. One notable resource is the ADA Consultant Dietitians in Health Care Facilities (CD-HCF) DPG. With a membership of 5,500, this group is a wealth of information. Members receive a quarterly newsletter, *The Consultant Dietitian,* and the DPG sells many excellent products including manuals and standards of practice. Refer to Chapter 9 for a listing of some of CD-HCF resources in this area.

Writing

Writing transcends most types of consulting. It is a component of most consulting positions. There are some consultants who make most of their income as authors. Opportunities for dietetics professionals seeking to earn income writing include the following:

- Writing educational materials or marketing pamphlets for companies to distribute either to the public or for professionals to use. They can also write educational materials to be sold to other professionals.
- Writing a book. Nutrition-related publications can be geared to the consumer or it can be a professional publication. Keep in mind, however, when writing for other professionals that you do narrow your market, thus decreasing potential revenue.
- Composing the nutrition component of manuals for health care facilities. For example, a dietetics professional can be contracted to write a nutrition chapter for a manual that would be used in a drug rehabilitation program.

- Technical writing for grants.
- Writing nutrition-related marketing materials for companies.
- Contributing to a much larger publication, such as a textbook or a parenting publication.

Consulting to the Media

The major media outlets are inundated with nutrition-related stories. Every time you pick up a women's, children's, family, health, beauty, or even a business magazine, there is some type of nutrition-related article. Nutrition remains a hot topic in the media. Dietetics professionals consult for the media in various capacities, such as the following:

- Serving as a consultant to a media outlet to validate the accuracy of information, either on or off air.
- Local cable shows will use dietetics professionals to perform cooking demonstrations or appear on talk shows.
- Write weekly columns for local newspapers.
- Write for major magazines. Professionals may write articles, monthly columns, or may perform recipe makeovers.

At times, you will be asked to do a media appearance or interview for free. These opportunities provide great exposure and therefore are wonderful marketing opportunities. Remember, the media is a constantly expanding source of potential opportunities.

Public Relations Firms

Food companies pay big bucks to promote their products. These companies hire public relations (PR) firms to market their products. More and more often, firms are looking to incorporate the nutrition expert into their campaigns. The PR firms are contracting with dietetics professionals to do the following:

- Lend credibility to a marketing campaign
- Write consumer education and marketing brochures
- Represent products at trade shows
- Conduct product demonstrations in malls or supermarkets
- Verify the accuracy of the nutritional content or the message of certain advertising campaigns

Many larger PR firms that represent food companies actually have a full time RD on staff. A great way to pursue spokesperson work is to send your biography and samples of your media work directly to that person.

If you do not have samples of media work, become active in your professional organizations to get contacts and begin building your media portfolio with local television, radio, or newspaper interviews. Your state dietetic association is a great place to start. Apply for the position of state media representative. This will pave the road to getting hired for spokesperson jobs.

If your goal is to become a spokesperson, you may want to set some ethical guidelines for yourself. It is always wise to determine in advance whether you have strong views about certain products. Make sure you believe in the product you will be promoting. Be true to yourself. Do not sell out! See Box 8.2 for information on how other dietetics professionals entered public relations.

BOX 8.2
SPOKESPERSON SUCCESS

Maye Musk, MS, RD

Maye Musk wanted to increase her media exposure. She sent out audition tapes and resumes to television stations, but to no avail. She then became active in dietetics organizations and met a fellow dietitian who worked in a public relations firm. Through this networking experience, she was soon contacted for a spokesperson position.

The public relations firm wanted her to represent a cottage cheese with added calcium. In her opinion, Ms. Musk felt her appeal was her age—she was in her mid-50s and the company's target market was postmenopausal women. The goal was to promote the benefits of calcium in reducing the risk of osteoporosis.

A contract and product "talking points" were sent to her. "Talking points" present the key message(s) the client wants to convey. The PR firm also provided a media training session, in which she practiced working the key message into her interviews. In this session they purposely attempted to take her off topic, to make sure she could handle difficult interviews.

Ms. Musk was then interviewed for the camera and scheduled for magazine interviews. She was flown to three cities to participate in health fairs and to provide media interviews. At the health fairs she was available to answer nutrition questions.

Hope Warshaw, MMSc, RD, CDE

Hope Warshaw was contacted by a public relations firm to represent a large national restaurant chain. They were launching a campaign to help educate consumers about eating healthier and smarter in their restaurant and in restaurants in general. The PR firm was referred to Hope through an RD colleague who works in the PR industry. Hope's colleague was familiar with her past publications and knew she was an expert on healthy restaurant eating. She also knew Hope had media spokesperson experience. After receiving approval from the restaurant chain, Ms. Warshaw was hired by the PR firm to conduct television, radio, and newspaper interviews on this topic.

(continues)

BOX 8.2 (continued)

Hope's advice to dietetics professionals seeking spokesperson work is to carefully evaluate the product or entity you are being asked to represent and the message you are being asked to provide. Make sure you are comfortable with both. Also, be careful not to take on too many accounts, to avoid overexposure with the media.

Pat Baird, RD

Pat Baird was selected by a public relations firm as a spokesperson for a company that was introducing a low-acid orange juice. The firm was familiar with one of her past publications, which featured a chapter on heartburn. For the spokesperson project, the target audience was adults who suffer from heartburn.

Ms. Baird worked on this project for about six months. Her activities included reviewing all press materials, including pitch letters and press releases, and reviewing all product information on low-acid juice. She also drafted an outline for a consumer booklet and acted as a liaison between the orange juice company and The National Heartburn Alliance. Additionally, she performed a television satellite media tour, a radio satellite media tour, and local TV and radio interviews.

Corporations

Studies have shown that healthy employees are more productive employees. Large companies like to be known as good companies to work for, and one way they can do so is by providing unique employee benefits. Employee wellness programs can meet both these needs. Companies that have employee wellness programs will often hire a dietetics professional to provide many of these services. They may contract an RD to

- teach classes such as brown-bag seminars. (Box 8.3 lists some sample topics for seminars.)
- write brochures or nutrition tips in employee newsletters.
- provide individual counseling.
- set up a group weight loss, diabetes, or cholesterol management program.
- consult with cafeterias to create healthy cafeteria menu items.

Some dietetics professionals make corporate wellness their primary source of revenue. This is quite a niche. If you have various corporate clients you can recycle your lessons, perhaps just tailoring them to the audience. You can even purchase ready-to-go seminars geared toward employee health and wellness. Many of them have been developed by successful corporate RDs.

BOX 8.3

TOPICS FOR SEMINARS OR CLASSES

- Eating on the run
- Healthy snacks
- Healthy restaurant meals
- Proper portions
- Fad diets
- Surviving the holidays
- Eating awareness
- Nutrition 101
- Weight management strategies
- Endurance eating
- Menopause myths
- Feeding your family
- Packing healthy lunches
- Alternative nutrition
- Carb loading
- Label reading
- Negotiating the grocery store
- Food safety

Fitness Centers

Glance through any newspaper and you will see that health clubs and gyms throughout the country are competing for members. They want to be able to offer as many services to their members as possible. Nutrition and fitness go hand in hand, so the opportunities for consulting work in these facilities abound. Dietetics professionals can capitalize on this fitness boom by offering the following services to a health club:

- Teaching classes to members. Team up with a personal trainer or good exercise instructor and create a package of services. It can be a series of classes or single topic classes. Perhaps the club can provide space to offer individual counseling to club members who request it.
- Write an article or provide nutrition "bites" for a newsletter or bulletin board.
- Provide a nutrition-related handout for the front desk.
- Set up an "Ask the Nutrition Expert Day" that will benefit members and increase your visibility.

Try to provide informational sessions with the trainers to get to know them. Inform them of your services and assure them you are not there to provide exercise advice. Because their clients tend to take their advice very seriously, trainers can affect your credibility greatly (either positively or negatively). Winning them over by demonstrating how you can complement them (not replacing them) is a real coup.

Consulting to health and fitness clubs presents unique payment issues. Some clubs may be willing to pay you as a consultant to provide elite services to their members. Too often, however, health clubs cannot afford that. They may request that you charge separately for your services. The challenge is to get the members to pay for extra services that are not included in their club membership. Although this sounds troubling, do not let it deter you. You may have to provide some free services in order to market yourself. It is possible to pitch your services to this venue. There are plenty of dietetics professionals who are successfully consulting to health and fitness clubs!

Physicians and Allied Health Practices

Some physicians and allied health practices find it beneficial to contract to have a registered dietitian on staff to work within various capacities, particularly if the physician's specialty area has a strong nutrition-related component. Endocrinologists who treat patients with diabetes, doctors who run weight management programs, or psychiatrists who treat patients with eating disorders are a few examples. They do not have the time to answer the many nutrition questions or provide the instruction that their patients seek, so they may contract with an RD to provide those services. Some dietetics professionals prefer this arrangement rather than having to deal with their own billing and other administrative duties. Often they are paid a consulting fee to see the patients that are scheduled for them, but the specifics could be worked out differently.

Sometimes a physician who has a "nutrition-related" practice will hire an RD as a consultant to perform administrative duties. One RD held a consulting position as the program coordinator of an eating-disorders program for a psychiatric practice. Her duties included talking to all potential patients over the phone; performing intake evaluations on all new patients to recommend a treatment plan; and marketing the program by speaking at schools, health fairs, employee assistance programs, and parenting groups. She was also responsible for placing advertisements in local newspapers.

Another RD once held a position as the nutrition education director of a large weight management program in a physician's office. Her duties included developing educational materials to give to patients and working with the staff nutritionists. If this type of position sounds appealing to you, try to target a practice that can use your expertise and go pitch your services. Tell them how your services can complement theirs.

Grocery Store Chains

Many large grocery store chains compete for the same consumer dollars, and they, too, want to be innovative in the services they provide. As consumers become more health conscious, these grocery store chains are implementing nutrition education programs and hiring dietetics professionals to develop and conduct these programs. Many of them rely on dietetics professionals to do the following:

- Write pamphlets and other marketing material in the form of nutrition handouts and recipes
- Provide grocery store tours
- Perform product and cooking demonstrations
- Work in the consumer relations departments

According to a survey published by the Food Marketing Institute, 6.2% of surveyed consumers' disposable income was spent on prepared foods (4). Consumers all want healthier options, even in prepared foods. An opportunity exists for the dietetics professional to develop these requested healthy items. Even local stores in small towns can use guest speakers and cooking demos, not to mention many of the other services mentioned. You can even purchase ready-to-go information on supermarket tours from several locations on the Internet.

A large grocery store chain in the Washington, DC, area encourages RDs to provide store tours and diabetes tours. In order to qualify to give the tours, the dietetics professional must be an RD, hold malpractice insurance, sign a "held harmless" agreement, and attend an orientation given by the company. The chain provides some training materials and information on how to market the tours. The RD is then free to contact the managers of individual stores to set up tours. It is a fabulous marketing opportunity. Check grocery store chains in your area for similar opportunities.

Consulting in Cyberspace

Dietetics professionals are writing for e-zines (online magazines), contributing the nutrition-related content to health education CDs, and writing content for technical and nontechnical nutrition-related sites. Some dietetics professionals have created excellent Web sites to provide public education and sell their products. Some provide online counseling to groups and individuals. Just like Cyberspace itself, this is a rapidly growing market for consultants. Chapter 7 provides more information on technology.

Beyond the Sky

There are simply too many other opportunities available to dietetics professionals to list them all. Think out of the proverbial box to create your own opportunities. See Box 8.4 for additional miscellaneous consulting venues for the dietetics professional.

BOX 8.4

POTENTIAL CONSULTING OPPORTUNITIES

- Alternative and complementary care practices

- Athletic teams

- Universities

- Restaurants

- Private schools

- Culinary schools

- Spas and day spas

- Camps

- Day-care centers

- Correctional institutions

- Group homes

- Dental offices

- Home health agencies

Whether you are consulting in a small capacity on a part-time basis or have big plans for developing a product or creating a large company employing other dietitians, you should now have some idea of the direction into which you want to expand your services.

Professional Examples

Now that we have explored some of the exciting and creative consulting venues available to dietetics professionals, we will highlight some dynamic, thriving entrepreneurs to give you a taste of what it is like to have your own business and work as a nutrition consultant. You may notice that these successful professionals describe their work in similar ways. Common threads exist, and perhaps you will recognize them as traits that constitute a successful entrepreneur. As you will see, successful entrepreneurs rarely put all their eggs in one basket; rather, they have multiple projects occurring simultaneously and the types of consulting vary regularly. Successful entrepreneurs are always thinking of the next project.

The following questions were posed to the expert entrepreneurs:

1. What do you call yourself?
2. What jobs do you do under the title of "consultant"?
3. What are your primary income sources?
4. How do you spend a typical day?
5. Please provide a description of your profession—perhaps a bio explaining what you do.

Toni Bloom, MS, RD

Ms. Bloom states that her cards do not list "nutritionist" or "dietitian," but they do show her MS, RD credentials. Her logo reads "nutrition counseling," "nutrition consulting," and "nutrition speaking." She feels it is more important that people know what she does rather than what they call her. When introducing herself at a speaking engagement, she refers to herself as both a registered dietitian and nutritionist, because she believes it is important that they understand the RD qualifications.

Ms. Bloom writes, creates menu plans, and works with chefs of wealthy clients to "fine-tune" their menu plans. She works with the county's employee health and fitness program to plan seminars, classes, and contests, such as weight loss or "Five a day," and she provides seminars to corporations.

Her biggest income sources are the individual clients she sees in her private practice, her job at the university teaching a sports nutrition class, and her county contract. The rest are all $500 to $5,000 "side jobs," which help pay the bills.

A typical day for Ms. Bloom consists of working in her home office from 6 or 7 A.M., checking e-mails until about 8 or 9 A.M. If she does not have an early appointment or class, she will go for a run and then get to one of her offices or the university or to a corporate client to give a talk. She prefers to have one day per week in which she does not have to go to the office so she can work in her home office on accounting, writing, projects, e-mail and "food coaching"—reviewing clients' food records via e-mail.

Ms. Bloom is the owner of Toni Bloom & Associates, a nutrition counseling and consulting firm with three offices in the San Francisco/Silicon Valley area. Toni received her master's degree in nutrition from Penn State and her bachelor's degree in nutrition/pre-medicine from Ohio University. She is the elected past chair of the ADA's Nutrition Entrepreneurs DPG. Toni's corporate client list includes Sun Microsystems and Hewlett Packard, and she's a resource for *Men's Health, Runner's World,* and NBC-TV/San Francisco.

Kathy Wise, RD

Ms. Wise places "Dietitian/Nutritionist" under her name on her business card. It is her opinion that outside the medical field the term "dietitian" can be a disadvantage. In her experience, the public relates to and understands the term "nutritionist." In her marketing materials, however, she uses the slogans "Your Personal Nutritionist" or "Your Nutrition Coach." Kathy provides one-on-one consulting for individuals, consults with businesses, and helps them develop programs and ideas to start and enhance their wellness programs. She serves as a consultant to an exercise equipment company and reviews or writes the nutrition information/diet that will be included with the piece of equipment.

Most of her income is from developing wellness programs and individual consultations. Requests for speaking engagements, which are much more lucrative than individual consultations, are increasing.

A sample day will start at 7:15 A.M., with a paid speaking engagement followed by individual client consultations in her office. Her day will end at about 6 P.M. Between clients, she will catch up on telephone calls and e-mails, and she will work on future programs and speaking engagements. Many corporate programs are scheduled for early morning or during the lunch hour, and speaking engagements are often at lunchtime or in the evening. One of her current contracts calls for her to provide a four-month weight loss and wellness series for a medical center.

Kathy has a partner, Robin K. Bowman, RD. They share a lot of work and brainstorm ideas. Kathy believes that getting her partner was one of the best things she did to expand her practice and save her sanity. She and her partner plan to focus this coming year on developing materials, programs, self-help workbooks, and journals for companies, schools, and individuals. They recognize that selling a product is imperative if they are going to survive and grow.

Ms. Wise's bio reads as follows: Kathy Wise, RD, LD, a member of The National Speakers Association, is a professional speaker and nutrition consultant to companies, physicians, schools and individuals. Every day she draws on her scientific expertise and sense of humor to make good nutrition fun, simple and meaningful for everyone. Ms. Wise works with local athletes and high school teams to help them perform at their optimal level. Another specialty area of Ms. Wise's is working with athletes with eating disorders.

Christine Palumbo, MBA, RD

Ms. Palumbo refers to herself as a nutrition communications consultant, a nutrition speaker, writer, and consultant. Ms. Palumbo has a diversified consulting business. As a freelance writer, she is the *Allure* magazine Food News columnist and a writer for FoodFit.com.

Christine speaks to corporations and in large hospital events on nutrition-related topics. She plans to continue to develop this aspect of her practice, because speaking is her passion. She performs nutrition analysis for magazines, books, PR firms, food companies, and restaurants.

Ms. Palumbo also maintains a private practice to keep in touch with what people are thinking. Ms. Palumbo teaches on a part-time basis at the local university and does some unpaid media work. She is a paid spokesperson for food companies and consults to PR firms, food companies, and commodity groups. Christine has always been in a volunteer position with ADA as well, either elected or appointed, because she thinks it is fun and helps her to stay "in the know."

Ms. Palumbo reports that in 2003, writing provided 32% of her income, spokesperson work 23%, nutrition analysis 19%, speaking 14%, consulting 7%, private practice 5%, and teaching 1%.

A sample day for Christine begins with reading e-mail first thing in the morning. She then takes her daughter to school, comes home and begins work at her desk. She may go out to exercise before beginning work or sometimes exercises midmorning.

Throughout the day, Christine checks her e-mail ("probably too often"). She thinks she could limit this more because e-mail becomes very enticing! She basically works on what the day's priority is or sometimes works on what she is in the mood for. At noon, she breaks for lunch, skims one of four newspapers she subscribes to, and then returns to her work. It is not uncommon for her to work at night or on weekends, sometimes seeing clients.

Ms. Palumbo has a diversified nutrition communications practice in which she writes, speaks, performs nutrition analysis, and provides nutrition counseling as well as paid spokesperson work.

Tracy Fox, MPH, RD

Ms. Fox generally refers to herself as a "Nutrition Policy Consultant." Her real title, however, is president of Food, Nutrition and Policy Consultants, LLC. Ms. Fox works on a variety of projects related to food and nutrition policy at the federal, state, and local levels.

She provides analysis and tracks federal policy issues related to nutrition and provides expertise to clients on how certain policies impact them and how they can impact policy. For example, she has been working with the Produce for Better Health Foundation in an effort to promote more fruits and vegetables in federal nutrition assistance programs, such as school lunch and WIC programs. Tracy speaks to health and nutrition audiences, including state and local health department professionals, on behalf of her clients on policy issues, especially in relation to promoting more fruits and vegetables through environmental and policy changes. She also provides advocacy training to teach health and nutrition professionals and others how to become better advocates. Ms. Fox meets with members of Congress and staff to lobby for health and nutrition issues. She is also working on a number of projects at the national and state levels to develop best practices for schools and school leaders to promote better nutrition and physical activity. These activities complement the numerous volunteer positions she holds at the county level that focus on improving beverage and food offerings in schools.

Ms. Fox's primary income sources come from private nonprofit companies, federal government agencies, other consultants and consulting companies, public relations firms and the food industry. When she is not traveling or in Washington, DC, she spends most of her day working in her home office.

Ms. Fox's bio reads as follows: Tracy Fox, president of Food, Nutrition & Policy Consultants, LLC has 20 years of experience working in the federal government and the private sector, and has extensive experience in federal nutrition policy and the legislative and regulatory process. Her clients include federal, state, and local agencies, public relations firms, food manufacturers, and nonprofit organizations where she provides advice and expertise on policy and nutrition initiatives. Ms. Fox is an advocate for children and dedicated to promoting healthy food and beverage choices in and out of school. Areas of expertise include child nutrition and school health, federal, state and local nutrition policy, advocacy and government relations.

Ms. Fox has been invited to speak by federal and state agencies as well as at the National Healthy School Summit. She has also presented at numerous professional association meetings and events. She is quoted regularly in media outlets on subjects including school nutrition, obesity, and federal nutrition policy.

Tammy Lakatos Shames, RD, CDN, CPT, and Lyssie Lakatos, RD, CDN, CPT

Ms. Lakatos Shames and Ms. Lakatos refer to themselves as registered dietitians. They provide corporate, group, and sports team seminars, as well as individual counseling. They write for various magazines and Web sites, appear in the media, and participate in health fairs. Ms. Lakatos Shames and Ms. Lakatos have multiple income sources, including a publication, individual consults, corporate seminars, and health fairs. A typical day begins with reviewing e-mails early in the morning, seeing clients, and attending fairs or providing seminars during the day. The day generally concludes by working on seminars or working on their book.

Tammy and Lyssie have quite a niche, just because they are twins in business together. Their bio reads as follows: Tammy Lakatos Shames and Elysse ("Lyssie") Lakatos share more than identical features; they share identical success in the competitive field of nutrition and wellness. Since relocating from Atlanta, Georgia, where they built a successful private practice with both individual and corporate clients, the twins have had stellar achievements in New York City.

In 1999 the Lakatoses joined the New York Health and Racquet Club to serve as nutritionist within the club, as well as corporate wellness nutritionists, attending health fairs and providing on-site nutrition lectures and nutrition consults at more than 200 corporations. In addition, Tammy and Lyssie were hired as the exclusive nutritionists for NBC's celebrities and employees at Rockefeller Plaza, and for Athlete International, a personal fitness company catering to elite, professional and weekend athletes. They also have helped train the U.S. "Eco-Challenge" team in preparation for the 24-hour competition, the top players on the Worldwide Senior Tennis Circuit, and participants in varied races and marathons.

The Lakatoses are the authors of a nutrition-related publication published by Simon and Schuster. They have been featured regularly as the nutrition experts on multiple major television broadcasting outlets and sought after contributors by many print and on-line publications.

Tammy and Lyssie have a private practice in New York City, where they counsel celebrities, athletes, and professionals and provide nutrition workshops for corporations.

Kate Geagan, MS, RD

Ms. Geagan refers to herself as a nutrition consultant. She is the codirector of IT Nutrition, a nutrition company she cofounded with her business partner in 2000. As a nutrition consultant, Ms. Geagan helps companies create effective nutrition programming, to keep their employees healthy and motivated. She also helps wellness companies offer innovative programs to their clients to help reduce health care costs.

Kate serves as a "nutrition expert" for a consulting firm—she is a consultant to companies who are looking to better understand consumer behaviors and the marketplace with regard to nutrition and their eating habits, helping these companies identify opportunities within their target market. She has also consulted for companies who are interested in working with the dietetics profession and are seeking to understand the RD's perspective. Ms. Geagan is currently working with the Massachusetts Department of Public Health to create and launch an effective program for police and fire stations statewide to address nutrition- and weight-related issues.

Ms. Geagan's primary income is provided by corporate seminars and spokesperson work. Every day is different and that is what Kate loves most about her job. Usually, she spends about 2 to 3 hours in the morning in her office following up on projects, beginning new projects, checking e-mails, and reading. Perhaps there are 3 to 5 hours of billable time on the road at seminars, consulting work, or a spokesperson engagement. She spends an average of one hour in meetings or conferences each day with her business partner or one of the groups or boards she is involved with. She often spends another hour or so developing future projects.

Ms. Geagan's bio is as follows: Kate Geagan MS, RD, is codirector of IT Nutrition, a nutrition consulting group specializing in corporate wellness programs, consulting and spokesperson work. Kate has worked with dozens of companies throughout Massachusetts to develop wellness seminars and counseling and weight loss programs for their employees, such as Sun Microsystems, Reebok International, Yankee Candle and Citistreet. She also works with numerous health care and wellness companies to provide nutrition services for their clients, such as Tufts Health Plan and Fitcorp.

Kate has worked extensively with the media as a spokesperson and a nutrition expert. She was the public relations chair for the Massachusetts Dietetic Association in 2002–2003, and has appeared on numerous television shows and news programs in the Boston market. In addition, Kate has worked with public relations firms such as Weber Shandwick on product launches and media tours in the Boston area. She has been quoted in the *Boston Globe, The Wall Street Journal,* and *Prevention* magazine, and wrote a nutrition column for the *Salem Evening News* from 2000 to 2002.

Nancy Collins, PhD, RD, CDN

Dr. Collins calls herself a consultant dietitian. Under the title of "consultant" she is an author, speaker, expert witness, medico-legal consultant, and a business development consultant to several major pharmaceutical firms and nutrition companies. She is also the director of nutrition for a nutrition technology company that develops interactive and personalized nutrition programs for corporate Web sites. In addition, Dr. Collins serves on several industry advisory and editorial panels, including the medical advisory board for the American Professional Wound Care Association and the editorial advisory boards of the journals *Advances in Skin and Wound* and *Extended Care Product News.* Most of Dr. Collins's income is generated from work related to her project development consulting, her position at the nutrition technology company, and her work as an expert witness.

Dr. Collins does not have a typical day—each day is different. A typical month will find her writing her column for the two journals in which she is featured, reviewing several medical charts for attorneys and probably testifying once at either a deposition or a trial. She will also be traveling out of town once or twice per month to speak at a conference or symposium, logging hours at the computer for her tech consulting, and working on a major project for a corporate client. Dr. Collins also devotes a portion of each week to activities that support the dietetics profession through her work with the Florida Dietetic Association and the American Dietetic Association. Her current role in the Florida Dietetic Association is director of information technology, and Dr. Collins also serves on the executive committee of the Nutrition Entrepreneurs DPG as newsletter editor.

Here is a description of Dr. Collins's work: Nancy Collins has operated her own consulting business for the past fifteen years. Although she started in long-term care, she now finds herself primarily engaged in national consulting. Dr. Collins's established expertise in several areas has led to various jobs. An accomplished author, she has written several book chapters, writes a nutrition question and answer column in a medical journal and a column for a magazine. Nancy has spoken at approximately 150 medical conferences and symposia across the country. She is an "expert witness" for cases involving long-term care malpractice with approximately 75 attorneys among her clients.

Dr. Collins consults to major pharmaceutical and medical nutrition companies and has worked on product launches, written white papers, monographs, marketing pieces, and Web site copy among other things. As the director of nutrition for a nutrition technology company, she provides services for Web-based nutrition applications that use the Internet. She is a past president of the Florida Dietetic Association and continues to be actively involved in professional issues. She is also the newsletter editor for the Nutrition Entrepreneurs DPG.

Are You Ready Now?

There are so many interesting, intense, innovative entrepreneurs across the country. The women highlighted above are only a few of the successful dietetic entrepreneurs. It was very difficult to decide which dietetics professionals to include. Hopefully, these examples inspired you. As you read these examples you should be able to glean some ideas that you can incorporate into your marketing plan. You can combine some or all or the various aspects of consulting to create your dream job. Now is the time for you to chart your course and control your career path.

The Sky's The Limit: A Summary

- Dietetics professionals nationwide are trading in their traditional jobs to start their own consulting businesses.
- Consulting and home-based businesses are a growing market trend. Economic downturns promote an increase in small home-based businesses.
- The benefits of self-employment in the field of dietetics include increased job satisfaction, scheduling flexibility, and higher salaries.
- The Internal Revenue Service has a list of criteria that determines whether someone is a consultant. A consultant has greater behavioral and financial control over the work they do—they make the decisions about how the work is done and are not reimbursed for expenses. Employee benefits are not provided to contractors.
- A dietetics professional in private practice provides individual and group nutrition counseling.
- Private practitioners often diversify and branch out into other areas of consulting, such as public speaking, writing, media and spokesperson work, health and fitness work, and corporate wellness.

References

1. Rogers D. Salary Survey Work Group. Report on the ADA 2002 dietetics compensation and benefits survey. *J Am Diet Assoc.* 2003;103:244–249.
2. Internal Revenue Service. *Employer's Supplemental Tax Guide.* Washington, DC: US Department of Treasury; 2004. IRS Publication 15A.
3. Herman R, Gioia J; the Herman Group. Microbusiness will offer economic strength [The Herman Group Web site]. April 9, 2003. Available at: http://www.herman.net/alert/archive_4-9-2003.html. Accessed March 2, 2004.
4. Food Marketing Institute. Supermarket facts—industry overview 2002. Available at: http://www.fmi.org/facts_figs/superfact.htm. Accessed December 15, 2003.

Chapter 9

Resources for Success

Publications for Starting and Staying in Business

The Everything Start Your Own Business Book: From Birth of Your Concept and Your First Deal, All You Need to Get Your Business Off the Ground, by Richard Mintzer. Avon, Mass: Adams Media Corporation, 2002.

The Girl's Guide to Starting Your Own Business: Candid Advice, Frank Talk, and True Stories for the Successful Entrepreneur, by Caitlin Friedman and Kimberly Yorio. New York, NY: HarperResource, 2003.

Small Business for Dummies, 2nd edition, by Eric Tyson and Jim Schell. New York, NY: Wiley Publishing, 2003.

Guerrilla Marketing: Secrets for Making Big Profits From Your Small Business, by Jay Conrad Levinson. Boston, Mass: Houghton Mifflin, 1998.

Working Solo: The Real Guide to Freedom and Financial Success with Your Own Business, by Terri Lonier. New York, NY: Wiley Publishing, 1998.

Be Your Own Boss Starter Kit, by Ann Litt and Faye Berger Mitchell (self-published).

Nutrition Resources and Products

Nutrient Analysis Software

Foodworks
The Nutrition Company
PO Box 477
Long Valley, NJ 07853
908/876-5580
http://www.nutritionco.com

The Food Processor
ESHA Research, Inc.
PO Box 13028
Salem, OR 97309
503/585-6242
http://www.esha.com

Nutribase
CyberSoft, Inc.
3851 East Thunderhill Place
Phoenix, AZ 85044
480/759-4849
http://www.nutribase.com

Organizations and Associations Providing Nutrition Education Resources

American Dietetic Association
120 South Riverside Plaza, Suite 2000
Chicago, IL 60606
800/877-1600
http://www.eatright.org

Dietetic Practice Groups of the American Dietetic Association
Members of the various practice groups receive free resources, such as monthly newsletters and access to electronic mailing lists. Most DPGs sell resources to both members and nonmembers. Consult their Web sites for further benefits (DPG sites are linked to the ADA Web site).

Key DPGs include the following:

- Nutrition Entrepreneurs (http://www.nedpg.org)
- Consultant Dietitians in Health Care Facilities (http://www.cdhcf.org)
- Dietitians in Business and Communications (http://www.dbconline.org)

Food and Health Communications
PO Box 266498
Weston, FL 33326
954/385-5328
http://www.foodandhealth.com

Food Allergy Network
11781 Lee Jackson Highway, Suite 160
Fairfax, VA 22033
800/929-4040
http://www.foodallergy.org

Gurze Books (educational resources on eating disorders)
PO Box 2238
Carlsbad, CA 92018
800/756-7533
http://www.bulimia.com

National Dairy Council
10255 West Higgins Rd, Suite 900
Rosemont, IL 60018
312/240-2880
http://www.nationaldairycouncil.org

Nasco Nutrition Teaching Aids
901 Janesville Ave
Fort Atkinson, WI 53538
800/558-9595
http://www.eNASCO.com

Nutrition Counseling Education Services Publications (NCES)
1904 E. 123rd St
Olathe, KS 66061
877/623-7266
http://www.ncescatalog.com

Produce for Better Health Foundation
5341 Limestone Rd
Wilmington, DE 19808
888/391-2100
http://www.5aday.com

The Vegetarian Resource Group (VRG)
PO Box 1463, Dept. IN
Baltimore, MD 21203
410/366-8343
http://www.vrg.org

Wheat Foods Council
10841 S Crossroads Dr, Suite 105
Parker, CO 80138
303/840-8787
http://www.wheatfoods.org

Newsletters and Periodicals

Dietetics professionals in private practice need to stay current and be well informed about general nutrition issues and topics of interest to patients. The following are newsletters and periodicals that write on hot topics and new trends.

American Institute for Cancer Research Newsletter
American Institute for Cancer Research
1759 R Street NW
Washington, DC 20009
800/843-8114
http://www.aicr.org
        Subscription is free; past issues online.

Consumer Health Digest
http://www.ncahf.org/digest/chd.html
        Free weekly e-mail newsletter, past issues archived and available online.

Cooking Light Magazine
PO Box 62376
Tampa, FL 33662
800/336-0125
www.cookinglight.com
        Periodical published eleven times per year; articles available online.

Eating Well: The Magazine for Food and Health
832A Ferry Road
Charlotte, VT 05445
802/425-5700
http://www.eatingwell.com
        Periodical published quarterly.

Environmental Nutrition
PO Box 420451
Palm Coast, FL
800/829-5384
http://www.environmentalnutrition.com
>Newsletter published twelve times per year.

FDA Consumer Magazine
Food and Drug Administration
5600 Fishers Lane
Rockville, MD 20857
888/463-6332
http://www.fda.gov/fdac
>Periodical published six times per year.

Harvard Health Letter
PO Box 420300
Palm Coast, FL 32142
800/829-9045
http://www.health.harvard.edu
>Monthly newsletter, past articles online for subscribers only.

Harvard Heart Letter
PO Box 420379
Palm Coast, FL 32142-0379
800/829-9171
http://www.health.harvard.edu

Harvard Women's Health Watch
PO Box 420068
Palm Coast, FL 32142-0068
800/829-5921
http://www.health.harvard.edu

Harvard Men's Health Watch
PO Box 421073
Palm Coast, FL 32142-1073
800/829-3341
http://www.health.harvard.edu

Mayo Clinic Health Letter
PO Box 531
Albert Lea, MN 56007
800/333-9037
http://www.mayohealth.org
> Eight-page monthly newsletter.

Nutrition Action Healthletter
1875 Connecticut Ave, NW, Suite 300
Washington, DC 20009
202/332-9110
http://www.cspinet.org
> Newsletter published ten times per year.

Today's Dietitian
3801 Schuylkill Road
Spring City, PA 19475
610/948-9500
http://www.todaysdietitian.com
> Periodical published twelve times per year.

Tufts University Health and Nutrition Letter
Tufts University Health and Nutrition
PO Box 420235
Palm Coast, FL 32142-0235
800/274-7581
http://www.healthletter.tufts.edu
> Newsletter published twelve times per year; abstracts available online.

UC Berkeley Wellness Letter
PO Box 420148
Palm Coast, FL 32142
386/447-6328
http://www.berkeleywellness.com
> Eight-page newsletter published twelve times per year.

Business Resources

Marketing

Food Marketing Institute Report
http://www.FMI.org.
> Annual research study that tracks consumer behavior and attitudes on a wide range of issues that are important to understanding the grocery shopper.

Marketresearch.com
http://www.marketresearch.com
    Compiles and sells market research reports by industry, market research publisher, and geographic area.

Trendwatching.com
http://www.trendwatching.com
    Focuses on consumer insights and behavioral trends, and the hands-on marketing/business opportunities they present. Provides a free monthly newsletter.

Consumer Trends Forum International
http://www.consumerexpert.org
    Nonprofit organization which, through newsletters and seminars, offers members information on consumer trends, networking resources, and perspectives into business solutions.

AllBusiness.com
http://www.allbusiness.com
    Provides numerous products and services, such as sample forms, contracts, and business plans, to small businesses.

Business Templates and Tools

Bplans.com
http://www.bplans.com
    Provides articles and links for creating successful business plans.

Startup Journal: The Wall Street Journal Center for Entrepreneurs
http://www.startupjournal.com
    Includes articles and templates for creating business plans.

Business Card Design, Marketing, and Printing Tips
http://www.businesscarddesign.com
    Includes links to templates, resources, and printers of business cards.

Nebs.com
http://www.nebs.com
    Source for personalized forms, invoices, and products for small businesses.

CCH Business Owner's Toolkit
http://www.toolkit.cch.com
    Provides information on starting, financing, and marketing your business.

Intuit QuickBooks
http://www.quickbooks.com
> Information on the popular accounting software QuickBooks.

General Business Support

US Small Business Association (SBA)
409 Third Street, SW
Washington, DC 20416
202/205-7701
http://www.sba.gov
> The SBA is a wealth of information for small businesses, providing assistance to help individuals start, run, and grow their businesses. Local SBAs may offer classes on specific topics.

Small Business Development Centers (SBDC)
http://www.sbaonlin.sba.gov/sbdc
> Sponsored by the SBA, the SBDC is staffed by former business owners who are available to help with your questions about small business.

The National Association for the Self-Employed (NASE)
PO Box 612067
DFW Airport
Dallas, TX 75261
800/232-6273
202/466-2100
http://www.nase.org
> Provides many benefits and services, including insurance and resources, to make small businesses successful.

Service Core of Retired Executives (SCORE)
409 3rd Street, SW, 6th Floor
Washington, DC 20024
800/634-0245
http://www.score.org
> A resource partner with the SBA that provides volunteers for small-business counseling.

Chamber of Commerce
http://www.2Chambers.com
> Nearly every town has a Chamber of Commerce. They can be helpful to small businesses in their communities.

My Own Business

http://www.MyOwnBusiness.com

Free online courses on starting a business.

FastTrac

http://www.FastTrac.org

Offers classes nationwide in starting and running small businesses.

Digital Women

http://www.digitalwomen.com

Provides free business resources and tools for women, including information on grants, home businesses, sales, and marketing.

COBRA Health Plan Advice for Individuals and Small Business

www.cobrahealth.com

Links and articles on health insurance for individuals and small businesses.

Insurance.com

http://www.insurance.com

Provides quotes on insurance.

Resources for Speakers

National Speakers Association (NSA)

1500 South Priest Dr

Tempe, AZ 85281

480/968-2552

http://www.nsaspeaker.org

Resources and education to advance the skills for those who speak professionally.

Toastmasters International Clubs

PO Box 9052

Mission Viejo, CA 92690

949/858-8255

http://www.toastmasters.org

A program that teaches individuals how to communicate effectively.

Government Resources

Internal Revenue Service
800/829-1040
http://www.irs.ustres.gov
For tax forms: http://www.irs.ustres.gov/forms
        For specific information on small businesses: http://www.irs.gov/business/small

National Center for Health Statistics
Office of Information Services
Hyattsville, MD 20782
301/458-4000
http://www.cdc.gov/nchs

National Health Information Center
PO Box 1133
Washington, DC 20013
800/336-4797
http://www.health.gov/nhic

Department of Health and Human Services
200 Independence Avenue, SW
Washington, DC 20201
877/696-6775
http://www.hhs.gov

Health Finder
c/o National Health Information Center
PO Box 1133
Washington, DC 20013-1133
http://www.healthfinder.gov

HIPAA Resources

HIPAA Guidelines

Office for Civil Rights—HIPAA
US Dept of Health and Human Services
http://www.hhs.gov/ocr/hipaa

Health Insurance Portability and Accountability Act of 1996
Centers for Medicare and Medicaid Services
http://www.cms.hhs.gov/hipaa/

HIPAA Obligations for Covered Entities
American Dietetic Association
http://www.eatright.org/member/policyinitiatives/83_11026.cfm
    ADA members-only Web site

HIPAA Regulations for Covered Entities
American Dietetic Association
http://www.eatright.org/member/policyinitiatives/83_17933.cfm
    ADA members-only Web site

Sample HIPAA Forms

Model HIPAA Notice of Privacy Practice
American Dietetic Association
http://www.eatright.org/member/files/hipaa040203b.doc
    ADA members-only Web site

Sample Patient Written Acknowledgement Confirming
Receipt of Privacy Notice
American Dietetic Association
http://www.eatright.org/Member
    ADA members-only Web site. (Search "Sample patient written
acknowledgement confirming receipt of privacy notice.")

MNT and Medicare Resources

Publications

*American Dietetic Association Medical Nutrition Therapy
Evidence-Based Guides for Practice*

- Chronic Kidney Disease (non-dialysis) Medical Nutrition Therapy
  Protocol CD-ROM
- Hyperlipidemia Medical Nutrition Therapy Protocol CD-ROM
- Nutrition Practice Guidelines for Gestational Diabetes Mellitus CD-
  ROM
- Nutrition Practice Guidelines for Type 1 and Type 2 Diabetes Mellitus
  CD-ROM

The Medicare MNT Provider
A monthly publication of ADA that provides timely Medicare and MNT advice, strategies, and articles.

Information

Medical Nutrition Therapy Links and Resources
American Dietetic Association
http://www.eatright.org/Member/83_12954.cfm
ADA members-only Web site

MNT State Carriers
American Dietetic Association
http://www.eatright.org/Member/PolicyInitiatives/statecarriers.cfm
ADA members-only Web site

CMS Form 1500 Questions and Answers
Centers for Medicare and Medicaid Services
http://www.boc.ca.gov/PubsVCP/CMS1500Q&A.pdf

CMS Form 1500 Health Claim Form
Centers for Medicare and Medicaid Services
http://www.cms.hhs.gov/providers/edi/cms1500.pdf

CMS Regional MNT Contacts
Centers for Medicare and Medicaid Services
http://www.cms.hhs.gov/about/regions/professionals.asp

ICD9 Database
Stanford University School of Medicine
http://neuro3.standford.edu/CodeWorrier

Appendix A

Model HIPAA Notice of Privacy Practices

HIPAA NOTICE OF PRIVACY PRACTICES

Effective Date: _____

THIS NOTICE DESCRIBES HOW PROTECTED HEALTH INFOR-MATION ABOUT YOU MAY BE USED AND DISCLOSED AND HOW YOU CAN GET ACCESS TO THIS INFORMATION. PLEASE REVIEW IT CAREFULLY.

If you have any questions about this notice, please contact:
[list clinic and privacy officer's name, title, address, phone, fax and e-mail (if applicable)]

OUR PLEDGE REGARDING PROTECTED HEALTH INFORMATION

We *[list name of clinic]* understand that protected health information about you and your health is personal. We are committed to protecting health information about you. This Notice applies to all of the records of your care generated by the *[list clinic name]*, whether made by *[list clinic name]* personnel or your personal doctor.

This Notice will tell you about the ways in which we may use and disclose protected health information about you. We also describe your rights and certain obligations we have regarding the use and disclosure of protected health information. The law requires us to:

- Make sure that protected health information that identifies you is kept private;

- Notify you about how we protect protected health information about you;
- Explain how, when and why we use and disclose protected health information;
- Follow the terms of the Notice that is currently in effect.

We are required to follow the procedures in this Notice. We reserve the right to change the terms of this Notice and to make new notice provisions effective for all protected health information that we maintain by:

- Posting the revised Notice in our office;
- Making copies of the revised Notice available upon request;
- Posting the revised Notice on our Web site.

HOW WE MAY USE AND DISCLOSE PROTECTED HEALTH INFORMATION ABOUT YOU

The following categories describe different ways that we use and disclose protected health information without your written authorization.

For Treatment. We may use protected health information about you to provide you with, coordinate or manage your medical treatment or services. We may disclose protected health information about you to doctors, nurses, technicians, medical students, or other *[insert clinic name]* personnel who are involved in taking care of you.

[Insert clinic name] staff may also share protected health information about you in order to coordinate the different things you need, such as prescriptions, lab work and x-rays. We also may disclose protected health information about you to people outside *[insert clinic name]* who may be involved in your medical care, such as clergy or others we use to provide services that are part of your care.

We may use and disclose protected health information to contact you as a reminder that you have an appointment for treatment or medical care at the *[insert clinic name]*. We may use and disclose protected health information to tell you about or recommend possible treatment options or alternatives or health-related benefits or services that may be of interest to you.

For Payment for Services. We may use and disclose protected health information about you so that the treatment and services you receive at the *[insert clinic name]* may be billed and payment may be collected from you, an insurance company or a third party. For example, we may need to give your health plan information about nutrition services you received at *[insert clinic's name]* so your health plan will pay us or reimburse you for the service. We may also tell your health plan about the nutrition services you are going to receive to obtain prior approval or to determine whether your plan will cover the treatment.

For Health Care Operations. We may use and disclose protected health information about you for *[insert clinic name]* health care operations, such as our quality assessment and improvement activities, case management, coordination of care, business planning, customer services and other activities. These uses and disclosures are necessary to run the facility, reduce health care costs, and make sure that all of our patients receive quality care.

For example, we may use protected health information to review our treatment and services and to evaluate the performance of the dietitian who is providing your services. We may also combine protected health information about many *[insert clinic name]* patients to decide what additional services the *[insert clinic name]* should offer, what services are not needed, and whether certain new treatments are effective. We may also disclose information to doctors, nurses, technicians, medical students, and other *[insert clinic name]* personnel for review and learning purposes. We may also combine the protected health information we have with protected health information from other health care facilities to compare how we are doing and see where we can make improvements in the care and services we offer. We may remove information that identifies you from this set of protected health information so others may use it to study health care and health care delivery without learning who the specific patients are. We may also contact you as part of a fundraising effort.

Subject to applicable state law, in some limited situations the law allows or requires us to use or disclose your health information for purposes beyond treatment, payment, and operations. However, some of the disclosures set forth below may never occur at our facilities.

As Required by Law. We will disclose protected health information about you when required to do so by federal, state or local law.

Research. We may disclose your PHI to researchers when their research has been approved by an institutional review board or privacy board that has reviewed the research proposal and established protocols to ensure the privacy of your information.

Health Risks. We may disclose protected health information about you to a government authority if we reasonably believe you are a victim of abuse, neglect or domestic violence. We will only disclose this type of information to the extent required by law, if you agree to the disclosure, or if the disclosure is allowed by law and we believe it is necessary to prevent or lessen a serious and imminent threat to you or another person.

Judicial and Administrative Proceedings. If you are involved in a lawsuit or dispute, we may disclose your information in response to a court or administrative order. We may also disclose health information about you in response to a subpoena, discovery request, or other lawful process by someone else involved in the dispute, but only if efforts have been made, either by us or the requesting party, to tell you about the request or to obtain an order protecting the information requested.

Business Associates. We may disclose information to business associates who perform services on our behalf (such as billing companies); however, we require them to appropriately safeguard your information.

Public Health. As required by law, we may disclose your protected health information to public health or legal authorities charged with preventing or controlling disease, injury, or disability.

To Avert a Serious Threat to Health or Safety. We may use and disclose protected health information about you when necessary to prevent a serious threat to your health and safety or the health and safety of the public or another person.

Health Oversight Activities. We may disclose protected health information to a health oversight agency for activities authorized by law. These activities include audits, investigations, and inspections, as necessary for licensure and for the government to monitor the health care system, government programs, and compliance with civil rights laws.

Law Enforcement. We may release protected health information as required by law, or in response to an order or warrant of a court, a subpoena, or an administrative request. We may also disclose protected health information in response to a request related to identification or location of an individual, victims of crime, decedents, or a crime on the premises.

Organ and Tissue Donation. If you are an organ donor, we may release protected health information to organizations that handle organ procurement or organ, eye or tissue transplantation or to an organ donation bank, as necessary to facilitate organ or tissue donation and transplantation.

Special Government Functions. If you are a member of the armed forces, we may release protected health information about you if it relates to military and veterans activities. We may also release your protected health information for national security and intelligence purposes, protective services for the President, and medical suitability or determinations of the Department of State.

Coroners, Medical Examiners, and Funeral Directors. We may release protected health information to a coroner or medical examiner. This may be necessary, for example, to identify a deceased person or determine the cause of death. We may also disclose protected health information to funeral directors consistent with applicable law to enable them to carry out their duties.

Correctional Institutions and Other Law Enforcement Custodial Situations.
If you are an inmate of a correctional institution or under the custody of a law
enforcement official, we may release protected health information about you
to the correctional institution or law enforcement official as necessary for your
or another person's health and safety.

Worker's Compensation. We may disclose information as necessary to comply with laws relating to worker's compensation or other similar programs
established by law.

Food and Drug Administration. We may disclose to the FDA, or persons
under the jurisdiction of the FDA, protected health information relative to
adverse events with respect to drugs, foods, supplements, products and product defects, or post marketing surveillance information to enable product
recalls, repairs, or replacement.

YOU CAN OBJECT TO CERTAIN USES AND DISCLOSURES

Unless you object, or request that only a limited amount or type of information be shared, we may use or disclose protected health information about you
in the following circumstances:

- We may share with a family member, relative, friend or other person
  identified by you protected health information directly relevant to
  that person's involvement in your care or payment for your care. We
  may also share information to notify these individuals of your location, general condition or death.
- We may share information with a public or private agency (such as the
  American Red Cross) for disaster relief purposes. Even if you object,
  we may still share this information if necessary for the emergency circumstances.

If you would like to object to use and disclosure of protected health
information in these circumstances, please call or write to our contact person
listed on page 1 of this Notice.

YOUR RIGHTS REGARDING PROTECTED
HEALTH INFORMATION ABOUT YOU

You have the following rights regarding protected health information we
maintain about you:

Right to Inspect and Copy. You have the right to inspect and copy protected
health information that may be used to make decisions about your care.
Usually, this includes medical and billing records.

To inspect and copy protected health information that may be used to make decisions about you, you must submit your request in writing to *[list clinic owner or privacy officer's name]*. If you request a copy of the information, we may charge a fee for the costs of copying, mailing or other supplies associated with your request, and we will respond to your request no later than 30 days after receiving it. There are certain situations in which we are not required to comply with your request. In these circumstances, we will respond to you in writing, stating why we will not grant your request and describe any rights you may have to request a review of our denial.

Right to Amend. If you feel that protected health information we have about you is incorrect or incomplete, you may ask us to amend or supplement the information.

To request an amendment, your request must be made in writing and submitted to *[list clinic owner or privacy officer's name]*. In addition, you must provide a reason that supports your request. We will act on your request for an amendment no later than 60 days after receiving the request.

We may deny your request for an amendment if it is not in writing or does not include a reason to support the request, and will provide a written denial to you. In addition, we may deny your request if you ask us to amend information that:

- Was not created by us, unless the person or entity that created the information is no longer available to make the amendment;
- Is not part of the protected health information kept by *[list clinic's name]*;
- Is not part of the information which you would be permitted to inspect and copy; or
- We believe is accurate and complete.

Right to an Accounting of Disclosures. You have the right to request an "accounting of disclosures." This is a list of the disclosures we made of protected health information about you.

To request this list or accounting of disclosures, you must submit your request in writing to *[list clinic owner or privacy officer's name]*. You may ask for disclosures made up to six years before your request (not including disclosures made before April 14, 2003). The first list you request within a 12-month period will be free. For additional lists, we may charge you for the costs of providing the list. We are required to provide a listing of all disclosures except the following:

- For your treatment
- For billing and collection of payment for your treatment
- For health care operations

- Made to or requested by you, or that you authorized
- Occurring as a byproduct of permitted use and disclosures
- For national security or intelligence purposes or to correctional institutions or law enforcement regarding inmates
- As part of a limited data set of information that does not contain information identifying you

Right to Request Restrictions. You have the right to request a restriction or limitation on the protected health information we use or disclose about you for treatment, payment or health care operations or to persons involved in your care.

We are not required to agree to your request. If we do agree, we will comply with your request unless the information is needed to provide you emergency treatment, the disclosure is to the Secretary of the Department of Health and Human Services, or the disclosure is for one of the purposes described in this document *[insert appropriate page numbers]*.

To request restrictions, you must make your request in writing to *[list clinic owner or privacy officer's name]*.

Right to Request Confidential Communications. You have the right to request that we communicate with you about medical matters in a certain way or at a certain location. For example, you can ask that we only contact you at work or by mail.

To request confidential communications, you must make your request in writing to *[list clinic owner or privacy officer's name]*. We will accommodate all reasonable requests.

Right to a Paper Copy of This Notice. You have the right to a paper copy of this Notice at any time by contacting *[list clinic owner or privacy officer's name]*.

OTHER USES AND DISCLOSURES

We will obtain your written authorization before using or disclosing your protected health information for purposes other than those provided for above (or as otherwise permitted or required by law). You may revoke this authorization in writing at any time. Upon receipt of the written revocation, we will stop using or disclosing your information, except to the extent that we have already taken action in reliance on the authorization.

YOU MAY FILE A COMPLAINT ABOUT OUR PRIVACY PRACTICES

If you believe your privacy rights have been violated, you may file a complaint with the *[insert clinic's owner or privacy officer's name]* or file a written complaint with the Secretary of the Department of Health and Human Services.

A complaint to the Secretary should be filed within 180 days of the occurrence or action that is the subject of the complaint.

If you file a complaint, we will not take any action against you or change our treatment of you in any way.

Appendix B

Code of Ethics for the Profession of Dietetics

The American Dietetic Association and its Commission on Dietetic Registration have adopted a voluntary, enforceable code of ethics. This code, entitled the Code of Ethics for the Profession of Dietetics, challenges all members, registered dietitians, and dietetic technicians, registered, to uphold ethical principles. The enforcement process for the Code of Ethics establishes a fair system to deal with complaints about members and credentialed practitioners from peers or the public.

The first code of ethics was adopted by the House of Delegates in October 1982; enforcement began in 1985. The code applied to members of the American Dietetic Association only. A second code was adopted by the House of Delegates in October 1987 and applied to all members and Commission on Dietetic Registration credentialed practitioners. A third revision of the code was adopted by the House of Delegates on October 18, 1998, and enforced as of June 1, 1999, for all members and Commission on Dietetic Registration credentialed practitioners.

The Ethics Committee is responsible for reviewing, promoting, and enforcing the Code. The Committee also educates members, credentialed practitioners, students, and the public about the ethical principles contained in the Code. Support of the Code of Ethics by members and credentialed practitioners is vital to guiding the profession's actions and to strengthening its credibility.

Preamble

The American Dietetic Association and its credentialing agency, the Commission on Dietetic Registration, believe it is in the best interest of the profession and the public it serves to have a Code of Ethics in place that provides guidance to dietetics practitioners in their professional practice and conduct. Dietetics practitioners have voluntarily adopted a Code of Ethics to reflect the values and ethical principles guiding the dietetics profession and to outline commitments and obligations of the dietetics practitioner to client, society, self, and the profession.

The Ethics Code applies in its entirety to members of the American Dietetic Association who are Registered Dietitians (RDs) or Dietetic Technicians, Registered (DTRs). Except for sections solely dealing with the credential, the Code applies to all members of The American Dietetic Association who are not RDs or DTRs. Except for aspects solely dealing with membership, the Code applies to all RDs and DTRs who are not members of the American Dietetic Association. All of the aforementioned are referred to in the Code as "dietetics practitioners." By accepting membership in the American Dietetic Association and/or accepting and maintaining Commission on Dietetic Registration credentials, members of the American Dietetic Association and Commission on Dietetic Registration credentialed dietetics practitioners agree to abide by the Code.

Principles

1. The dietetics practitioner conducts himself/herself with honesty, integrity, and fairness.
2. The dietetics practitioner practices dietetics based on scientific principles and current information.
3. The dietetics practitioner presents substantiated information and interprets controversial information without personal bias, recognizing that legitimate differences of opinion exist.
4. The dietetics practitioner assumes responsibility and accountability for personal competence in practice, continually striving to increase professional knowledge and skills and to apply them in practice.
5. The dietetics practitioner recognizes and exercises professional judgment within the limits of his/her qualifications and collaborates with others, seeks counsel, or makes referrals as appropriate.
6. The dietetics practitioner provides sufficient information to enable clients and others to make their own informed decisions.
7. The dietetics practitioner protects confidential information and makes full disclosure about any limitations on his/her ability to guarantee full confidentiality.
8. The dietetics practitioner provides professional services with objectivity and with respect for the unique needs and values of individuals.

9. The dietetics practitioner provides professional services in a manner that is sensitive to cultural differences and does not discriminate against others on the basis of race, ethnicity, creed, religion, disability, sex, age, sexual orientation, or national origin.

10. The dietetics practitioner does not engage in sexual harassment in connection with professional practice.

11. The dietetics practitioner provides objective evaluations of performance for employees and coworkers, candidates for employment, students, professional association memberships, awards, or scholarships. The dietetics practitioner makes all reasonable effort to avoid bias in any kind of professional evaluation of others.

12. The dietetics practitioner is alert to situations that might cause a conflict of interest or have the appearance of a conflict. The dietetics practitioner provides full disclosure when a real or potential conflict of interest arises.

13. The dietetics practitioner who wishes to inform the public and colleagues of his/her services does so by using factual information. The dietetics practitioner does not advertise in a false or misleading manner.

14. The dietetics practitioner promotes or endorses products in a manner that is neither false nor misleading.

15. The dietetics practitioner permits the use of his/her name for the purpose of certifying that dietetics services have been rendered only if he/she has provided or supervised the provision of those services.

16. The dietetics practitioner accurately presents professional qualifications and credentials.

    a. The dietetics practitioner uses Commission on Dietetic Registration awarded credentials ("RD" or "Registered Dietitian"; "DTR" or "Dietetic Technician, Registered"; "CSP" or "Certified Specialist in Pediatric Nutrition"; "CSR" or "Certified Specialist in Renal Nutrition"; and "FADA" or "Fellow of The American Dietetic Association") only when the credential is current and authorized by the Commission on Dietetic Registration. The dietetics practitioner provides accurate information and complies with all requirements of the Commission on Dietetic Registration program in which he/she is seeking initial or continued credentials from the Commission on Dietetic Registration.

    b. The dietetics practitioner is subject to disciplinary action for aiding another person in violating any Commission on Dietetic Registration requirements or aiding another person in representing himself/herself as Commission on Dietetic Registration credentialed when he/she is not.

17. The dietetics practitioner withdraws from professional practice under the following circumstances:
    a. The dietetics practitioner has engaged in any substance abuse that could affect his/her practice;
    b. The dietetics practitioner has been adjudged by a court to be mentally incompetent;
    c. The dietetics practitioner has an emotional or mental disability that affects his/her practice in a manner that could harm the client or others.
18. The dietetics practitioner complies with all applicable laws and regulations concerning the profession and is subject to disciplinary action under the following circumstances:
    a. The dietetics practitioner has been convicted of a crime under the laws of the United States which is a felony or a misdemeanor, an essential element of which is dishonesty, and which is related to the practice of the profession.
    b. The dietetics practitioner has been disciplined by a state, and at least one of the grounds for the discipline is the same or substantially equivalent to these principles.
    c. The dietetics practitioner has committed an act of misfeasance or malfeasance which is directly related to the practice of the profession as determined by a court of competent jurisdiction, a licensing board, or an agency of a governmental body.
19. The dietetics practitioner supports and promotes high standards of professional practice. The dietetics practitioner accepts the obligation to protect clients, the public, and the profession by upholding the Code of Ethics for the Profession of Dietetics and by reporting alleged violations of the Code through the defined review process of the American Dietetic Association and its credentialing agency, the Commission on Dietetic Registration.

Consideration of Ethics Issues

Committee

A 3-person committee, comprised of members of the American Dietetic Association and/or Commission on Dietetic Registration credentialed practitioners, will be appointed to handle all ethics matters. One person will be appointed each by the President of the American Dietetic Association, the Chairperson of the Commission on Dietetic Registration, and the Speaker of the House of Delegates. Terms of office will be for 3 years. Initial terms will be staggered to allow for continuity. The American Dietetic Association

President's initial appointment will serve for 3 years; the Chairperson of the Commission on Dietetic Registration's initial appointment will serve for 2 years; and the Speaker of the House of Delegates' initial appointment will serve for 1 year. Thereafter, each appointee will serve for 3 years. The chairmanship will rotate among the 3 Committee members. The American Dietetic Association President's appointment will serve first as chair followed in sequence by the Commission on Dietetic Registration Chairperson's and the HOD Speaker's appointments.

The Committee will have authority to consult with subject experts as necessary to conduct its business. The Committee may perform such other educational activities as might be necessary to assist members and credentialed individuals to understand the Code of Ethics.

Ethics Opinions

The Committee may issue opinions on ethics issues under the Code on its own initiative or in response to a member's or credentialed practitioner's request. These opinions will be available to members and credentialed practitioners to guide their conduct and to the public. Situations may be factual or hypothetical, but no names will be disclosed.

Ethics Cases

PREAMBLE

The enforcement procedures are intended to permit a fair resolution of disputes on ethical practices in a manner that protects the rights of individuals while promoting understanding and ethical practice. The Ethics Committee has the authority and flexibility to determine the best way to resolve a dispute, including educational means where appropriate.

1. COMPLAINT

A complaint that a member or credentialed practitioner has allegedly violated the Code of Ethics for the Profession of Dietetics must be submitted in writing on the appropriate form to the Ethics Committee.

The complaint must be made within 1 year of the date that the complainant (person making complaint) first became aware of the alleged violation or within 1 year from the issuance of a final decision in an administrative, licensure board, or judicial action involving the facts asserted in the complaint.

The complainant need not be a member of the American Dietetic Association or a practitioner credentialed by the Commission on Dietetic Registration.

The complaint must contain details on the activities complained of; the basis for complainant's knowledge of these activities; names, addresses, and telephone numbers of all persons involved or who might have knowledge of the activities; and whether the complaint has been submitted to a court, an administrative body, or a state licensure board. The complaint must also cite the section(s) of the Code of Ethics for the Profession of Dietetics allegedly violated.

The complaint must be signed and sworn to by the complainant(s).

2. PRELIMINARY REVIEW OF COMPLAINT

The chair of the Ethics Committee, legal counsel for the American Dietetic Association, and appropriate staff will review the complaint to determine if all the required information has been submitted by the complainant and whether an ethics question is involved.

If a complaint is made regarding an alleged violation of the Code of Ethics for the Profession of Dietetics and a similar complaint is already under consideration regarding the same individual by a state licensure board of examiners, an administrative body, or a court of law, the Ethics Committee will not process the complaint until a final decision has been issued.

3. RESPONSE

If the persons making the preliminary review determine that the process should proceed, the chair of the Ethics Committee will notify the respondent (person against whom the complaint is made) that a complaint has been made.

The notice will be sent from the staff via certified mail, return-receipt requested. The respondent will be sent a copy of the complaint, the Code of Ethics for the Profession of Dietetics, the Review Process, and Response to Complaint form.

The respondent will have thirty (30) days from receipt of the notification in which to submit a response. The response must be signed and sworn to by the respondent(s).

If the Ethics Committee does not receive a response, the chair of the Ethics Committee or his/her designee will contact the respondent by telephone. If contact with the respondent is still not made, a written notice will be sent. Failure to reach the respondent will not prevent the Committee from proceeding with the investigation.

4. ETHICS COMMITTEE REVIEW

If the chair of the Ethics Committee deems it appropriate, after consultation with legal counsel and appropriate staff, he/she will submit the complaint and the response to the Ethics Committee for review.

The Committee has broad discretion to determine how to proceed, including, but not limited to, dismissing the complaint, requesting further information from the parties, resolving the case through educational activities, holding a hearing as specified hereafter, or in any other way deemed advisable. The Committee may use experts to assist it in reviewing the complaint and response and determining further action.

At the appropriate time, the Ethics Committee will notify the complainant and the respondent of its decision, which may include the Committee's preliminary opinion with a request that the respondent take certain actions, including, but not limited to, successful completion of continuing professional education in designated areas, or supervised practice on terms to be set forth by the Committee.

The Ethics Committee may also recommend appropriate remedial action to the parties, which if undertaken, would resolve the matter.

The Ethics Committee may recommend, in its discretion, that a hearing be held subject to the other provisions of these procedures.

5. LICENSURE BOARD ACTION OR FINAL JUDICIAL OR ADMINISTRATIVE ACTION

When the Ethics Committee is informed by a state licensure body that a person subject to the Code of Ethics for the Profession of Dietetics has had his/her license suspended or revoked for reasons covered by the Code, the Committee may take appropriate disciplinary action without a formal hearing.

When a person has been finally adjudged or has admitted to committing a misdemeanor or felony as specified in Principle 18 of the Code, the Committee may take appropriate disciplinary action without a formal hearing.

6. HEARINGS

A. General   Hearings shall be held as determined by the Ethics Committee under the following guidelines. Hearing dates will be established by the chairman of the Ethics Committee. All hearings will be held in Chicago.

The Ethics Committee will notify the respondent and the complainant by certified mail, return-receipt requested, of the date, time, and place of the hearing.

The respondent may request a copy of the file on the case and will be allowed at least one postponement, provided the request for postponement is received by the American Dietetic Association at least fourteen (14) days before the hearing date.

B. Conduct of Hearings   The chair of the Ethics Committee will conduct a hearing with appropriate staff and legal counsel present. Individuals who have no conflict of interest will be appointed.

In the event that any Ethics Committee member cannot serve on the hearing panel for any reason, a replacement will be appointed by the representative of the original body that made the appointment, either the American Dietetic Association President, the Commission on Dietetic Registration Chairperson, or the Speaker of the House of Delegates as appropriate.

The parties shall have the right to appear; to present witnesses and evidence; to cross-examine the opposing party and adverse witnesses; and to have legal counsel present. Legal counsel for the parties may advise their clients, but may only participate in the hearings with the permission of the chair.

The hearing is the sole opportunity for the participants to present their positions.

Three members of the Ethics Committee shall constitute a quorum. Affirmative vote of two-thirds (2/3) of the members voting will be required to reach a decision.

A transcript will be prepared and will be available to the parties at cost.

C. Costs   The American Dietetic Association will bear the costs for the Ethics Committee, legal counsel, staff, and any other parties called by the American Dietetic Association. The American Dietetic Association will bear the travel and one night's hotel expenses for the complainant and respondent and one person that each chooses to bring, provided that such person is necessary to the conduct of the hearing as determined by the Chair of the Ethics Committee. The Ethics Committee shall issue regulations to govern the payment of these expenses which shall be incorporated and made part of these procedures.

The respondent and the complainant will be responsible for all costs and fees incurred in their preparation for and attendance at the hearing, except expenses for travel and hotel as stated above.

D. Decision   The Ethics Committee will render a written decision specifying the reasons therefor and citing the provision(s) of the Code of Ethics for the Profession of Dietetics that may have been violated. The Committee will decide that:

1. The respondent be acquitted;
2. Educational opportunities be pursued;
3. The respondent be censured, placed on probation, suspended, or expelled from the American Dietetic Association; and/or

4. The credential of the respondent be suspended or revoked by the Commission on Dietetic Registration of the American Dietetic Association.

The decision of the Ethics Committee will be sent to the respondent and the complainant as soon as practicable after the hearing.

7. DEFINITIONS OF DISCIPLINARY ACTION

Censure: A written reprimand expressing disapproval of conduct. It carries no loss of membership or registration status, but may result in removal from office at the national, state, and district levels and from committee membership. Time frame—not applicable.

Probation: A directive to allow for correction of behavior specified in Principle 17 of the Code of Ethics for the Profession of Dietetics. It may include mandatory participation in remedial programs (eg, education, professional counseling, peer assistance). Failure to successfully complete these programs may result in other disciplinary action being taken. It carries no loss of membership or registration status, but may result in removal from office at the national, state, and district levels and from committee membership. Time frame—specified time to be decided on a case-by-case basis.

Suspension: Temporary loss of membership and all membership benefits and privileges for a specified time with the exception of retention of coverage under health and disability insurance. The American Dietetic Association group malpractice insurance will not be available and will not be renewed during the suspension period. Time frame—specified time to be decided on a case-by-case basis.

Suspension of Registration: Temporary loss of credential and all benefits and privileges for a specified period of time. It may include mandatory participation in remedial programs (eg, education, professional counseling, peer assistance).

At the end of the specified suspension period, membership and registration benefits and privileges are automatically restored. Time frame—specified time to be decided on a case-by-case basis.

Expulsion: Removal from membership and a loss of all benefits and privileges. Time frame—may apply for reinstatement after a 5-year period has elapsed or sooner if the basis for the expulsion has been removed, with payment of a reinstatement fee. Must meet membership requirements in effect at the time of application for reinstatement.

Revocation of Credential: Loss of registration status and removal from registry; loss of all benefits and privileges. Upon revocation, the former credentialed practitioner shall return the registration identification card to the

Commission on Dietetic Registration. Time frame—Specified time for reapplication to be decided on a case-by-case basis, but, at a minimum, current recertification requirements would need to be met. A credential will not be issued until the Commission on Dietetic Registration determines that the reasons for revocation have been removed.

8. APPEALS

A. General   Only the respondent may appeal an adverse decision to the American Dietetic Association. During the appeals process, the membership and registration status of the respondent remains unchanged.

The American Dietetic Association President, the Chairperson of the Commission on Dietetic Registration, and the Speaker of the House of Delegates shall each appoint one person to hear the appeal. These individuals shall constitute the Appeals Committee for that particular case. Individuals who have no conflict of interest will be appointed.

B. Recourse to the Appeals Committee   To request a hearing before the Appeals Committee, the respondent/appellant shall notify the appropriate staff at the American Dietetic Association headquarters, by certified mail, return-receipt requested, that the respondent wishes to appeal the decision. This notification must be received within thirty (30) calendar days after receipt of the letter advising the respondent/appellant of the Ethics Committee's decision.

C. Contents   The appeal must comply with the following:

1. The appeal must be in writing and contain, at a minimum, the following information:
   a. The decision being appealed
   b. The date of the decision
   c. Why the individual feels the decision is wrong or was improperly rendered (See 8, E, "Scope of Review," below)
   d. The redress sought by the individual
   e. The appeal will be signed and sworn to.

If the appeal does not contain the information listed above, it will be returned to the individual, who will be given ten (10) calendar days to resubmit. Failure to furnish the required information within ten (10) calendar days will result in the appeal being waived.

D. Procedures   Upon receipt of this notification, appropriate staff shall promptly notify the chair of the Appeals Committee that the respondent/appellant is appealing a decision made by the Ethics Committee.

The Appeals Committee chair shall acknowledge the appeal and request a copy of the relevant written information on the case from appropriate staff.

1. *Location and participants*
   a. All appeals hearings will be held in Chicago.
   b. The complainant/appellee, the respondent/appellant, and the chair of the Ethics Committee will have the opportunity to participate in the appeals hearing.
   c. The parties may have legal counsel present, who may advise their clients, but may only participate in the hearings with the permission of the chair.
   d. Attendance at the hearing will be limited to persons determined by the chair to have a direct connection with the appeal and appropriate staff and legal counsel.
2. *Conduct of the hearing*   The three parties involved in the appeal will be given the opportunity to state why the decision and/or disciplinary action of the Ethics Committee should be upheld, modified, or reversed.

E. Scope of Review   The Appeals Committee will determine whether the Ethics Committee committed procedural error that affected its decision, whether the Ethics Committee's decision was contrary to the weight of the evidence presented to it, or whether there is new and substantial evidence that would likely have affected the Ethics Committee's decision that was unavailable to the parties at the time of the Ethics Committee's hearing for reasons beyond their control.

In reviewing the decision of the Ethics Committee, the Appeals Committee shall consider only the transcript of the hearing and the evidence presented to the Ethics Committee.

F. Record of Hearing   A transcript will be prepared and will be maintained in the case file.

G. Decision of Appeals Committee
   1. The Appeals Committee shall prepare a written decision stating the reasons therefor. The decision shall be to affirm, modify, or reject the decision and/or disciplinary action of the Ethics Committee or to remand the case to the Ethics Committee with instructions for further proceedings.
   2. Decisions of the Appeals Committee will be final.

H. Costs   The American Dietetic Association will bear the costs for the Appeals Committee, staff and legal counsel, and any parties called by the American Dietetic Association. The American Dietetic Association will bear the travel and one night's hotel expenses for the respondent/appellant, the complainant/appellee, and the chair of the Ethics Committee. The Ethics Committee shall issue regulations to govern the payment of these expenses, which shall be incorporated and made part of this procedure.

The respondent/appellant and the complainant/appellee will be responsible for all costs and fees incurred in their preparation for and attendance at the hearing, except expenses for travel and hotel as stated above.

9. NOTIFICATION OF ADVERSE ACTION

If the respondent is disciplined by the Ethics Committee and does not appeal the decision, the chair of the Ethics Committee will notify the appropriate American Dietetic Association organizational units, Commission on Dietetic Registration, the affiliate dietetic association, appropriate licensure boards, and governmental and private bodies within thirty (30) days after notification of the final decision.

In the event the respondent appeals a decision to discipline him/her and the Ethics Committee decision is affirmed or modified, similar notification will be made by the chair of the Ethics Committee.

In response to an inquiry about registration status, the Office on Dietetic Credentialing will state only whether a person is currently registered.

10. RECORDKEEPING

A. Records will be kept for a period of time after the disposition of the case in accordance with the American Dietetic Association's record retention policy.
B. Information will be provided only upon written request and affirmative response from the American Dietetic Association's legal counsel.

11. CONFIDENTIALITY PROCEDURES

The following procedures have been developed to protect the confidentiality of both the complainant and the respondent in the investigation of a complaint of an alleged violation of the Code of Ethics for the Profession of Dietetics:

A. The need for confidentiality will be stressed in initial communications with all parties.
B. Committee members will refrain from discussing the complaint and hearing outside of official committee business pertaining to the complaint and hearing.
C. If the hearing on a complaint carries over to the next Committee, the complaint will be heard by the original Committee to hear the complaint.

D. Communication with American Dietetic Association witnesses will be the responsibility of the Committee chair or staff liaison.

E. Witnesses who testify on behalf of The American Dietetic Association will be informed of the confidentiality requirements and agree to abide by them.

F. The Committee chair will stress the importance of confidentiality at the time of the hearing.

G. To ensure confidentiality, the only record of the hearing will be the official transcript and accompanying materials which will be kept at The American Dietetic Association offices. All other materials that were mailed or distributed to committee members should be returned to The American Dietetic Association staff, along with any notes taken by Committee members.

H. The transcript will be available if there is an appeal of the Ethics Committee's decision and only to the parties, Ethics Committee members, Appeals Committee members, The American Dietetic Association legal counsel, and staff directly involved with the appeal.

Index

About the Authors

Ann S. Litt, MS, RD

In private practice since 1980, Ann Litt, MS, RD, specializes in helping teenagers and young adults develop normal eating habits. She is the cocreator of the *Be Your Own Boss—The Basics of Starting a Private Practice* workshops, which have been presented to dietitians throughout the United States for more than ten years.

Litt is the author of *The College Student's Guide to Eating Well on Campus* (Tulip Hill Press, 2000) and *Fuel for Young Athletes* (Human Kinetics, 2004) and writes or is quoted regularly in the *Washington Parent* and the *Washington Post*. In addition, she is a nutrition consultant to the Washington Redskins.

She is presently a Professional Issues Delegate for Consultation and Business Practice in the American Dietetic Associations House of Delegates, is a past chairperson of Nutrition Entrepreneurs Dietetic Practice Group, and was the recipient of the Recognized Young Dietitian Award from the ADA.

Litt lives outside of Washington, DC, with her husband and two teenage sons.

Faye Berger Mitchell, RD

For 16 years Faye Berger Mitchell, RD, has assisted clients attain normal eating and healthy weight. She specializes in eating disorders treatment, women's nutrition, and weight management.

A spokesperson, a consultant in a variety of settings, and a support group facilitator, Berger Mitchell is frequently quoted in the *Washington Post* and *USA Today*. She also hosted *Nutrition Now* a biweekly television spot on cable evening news.

Berger Mitchell shares her experience and knowledge in private practice as cocreator of the *Be Your Own Boss—The Basics of Starting a Private Practice* workshops, which are presented to dietitians nationwide and provide guidance on how to start and maintain a private practice. In addition, she provides individual consultation to dietitians across the country to help them establish their practices. She has been a speaker at state and regional dietetic association meetings and has presented at several American Dietetic Association meetings.

Berger Mitchell's accomplishments have been acknowledged with a Recognized Young Dietitian Award from the ADA.

When not busy with her work, Berger Mitchell is at home with her husband in Washington, DC, or carpooling her two young, energetic daughters.